Disorders of Human Communication 4

Edited by G. E. Arnold, F. Winckel, B. D. Wyke

J. A. M. Martin

Voice, Speech, and Language in the Child: Development and Disorder

Springer-Verlag Wien GmbH

John Antony Michael Martin, M.B., B.S., F.R.C.S.

Director, Nuffield Hearing and Speech Centre and Consultant in Audiological Medicine, Royal National Throat, Nose and Ear Hospital; Honorary Research Fellow, Department of Phonetics and Linguistics, University College, London, Great Britain

Originally published by Springer-Verlag/Wien in 1981
Softcover reprint of the hardcover 1st edition 1981

With 43 Figures

ISSN 0173-170X

ISBN 978-3-7091-7044-1 ISBN 978-3-7091-7042-7 (eBook)
DOI 10.1007/978-3-7091-7042-7

Editors' Foreword

This volume is one in a series of monographs being issued under the general title of "Disorders of Human Communication". Each monograph deals in detail with a particular aspect of vocal communication and its disorders, and is written by internationally distinguished experts. Therefore, the series will provide an authoritative source of up-to-date scientific and clinical information relating to the whole field of normal and abnormal speech communication, and as such will succeed the earlier monumental work "Handbuch der Stimm- und Sprachheilkunde" by R. Luchsinger and G. E. Arnold (last issued in 1970). This series will prove invaluable for clinicians, teachers and research workers in phoniatrics and logopaedics, phonetics and linguistics, speech pathology, otolaryngology, neurology and neurosurgery, psychology and psychiatry, paediatrics and audiology. Several of the monographs will also be useful to voice and singing teachers, and to their pupils.

G. E. Arnold, Jackson, Miss.
F. Winckel, Berlin
B. D. Wyke, London

Since it was their chatter which prompted the question, this book is dedicated to Sarah and Vicky; to Peter who provided some of the answers; to Dorothy in gratitude; and to Him who in the beginning was the Word.

Preface

These pages are the long-delayed product of questions prompted by the spontaneous chatter of my two daughters when they were little. It was only possible to begin to explore these unformed thoughts through the repeated kindness of medical friends who allowed me to record their new-born children. Concomitant with the arrival of our son we moved to Kampala where I was able to record the children of African, Asian and English origin and my thanks are due to all these families for their unvarying friendliness, interest and help. Those children whose voices are not portrayed in Chapter 4 are no less important for the information they provided so that a more general and comprehensive picture of the development of the first stages of speech could emerge.

Whilst working in Mulago Hospital the large numbers of severely deaf children began to demand attention, and through the special clinics which this work necessitated, the existence of other forms of language disorder came unexpectedly to light. It subsequently became possible to relinquish active practice in ear, nose and throat surgery and turn to the problems of diagnosis, assessment and management of these children. In this I have been greatly helped by so many colleagues, both on the staff of the Nuffield Hearing and Speech Centre and elsewhere, that it is not possible to include all the doctors, teachers of the deaf, nursery teachers, psychologists, physicists and speech therapists by name. Their expertise, discussion and advice have been essential and I owe them a debt of gratitude which can only be repaid in the way they would choose, through attempts to achieve a deeper understanding of the specific problems and needs of these children. Amongst so many, particular mention must be made of the insights and assistance of the late Dr. M. Sheridan, Mr. H. A. Beagley, Miss P. Denny, Dr. R. Conrad, Dr. D. Kemp, Dr. J. Knight, Professor J. Colley, Dr. W. Moore, Professor D. Harrison, Professor D. Crystal, Professor A. Fourcin, Dr. J. Reynell, Mrs. C. Wright, Miss J. Harrison, Miss R. Warde, Mrs. D. Aly Khan, Miss P. Colyer and Miss V. Williamson. As representatives of the many speech therapists without whose help the clinical work would not have been possible mention must be made of Miss P. Griffiths, Miss S. Smith, Mrs. E. Paul, Miss V. Savage and especially Miss V. Connery.

I must thank the U.K. Editor of this series on "Disorder of Human Communication", Dr. Barry Wyke for giving me the opportunity and encouragement to commit my ideas and observations to paper, and so affording me the privilege of following in the footsteps of Luchsinger and Arnold's major work, "Voice, Speech and Language". My thanks are due to the board of Governors of the Royal National Throat, Nose and Ear Hospital and to the House Governor, Mr. G. Fulcher for facilitating the path of a full-time clinician who unwisely puts pen to paper, to Mr. D. Connolly and his staff for photographic assistance, and to Miss Mary Miller for her typing. My wife Dorothy not only produced some of the raw material, but prepared the initial analyses of the recordings of normal vocal development and of the details of clinical language disorder; without her the book would never have been written.

London, May 1981 **J. A. M. Martin**

Acknowledgement is gratefully made to a number of publishers and authors for permission to include quotations or to reproduce figures from their works: Cambridge University Press, Journal of Child Language, April 1975, Table 1, page 31, from "Holophrases, speech acts and language universals" by J. Dore; Fontana Paperbacks (W. Collins Sons & Co. Ltd.), quotations of extracts from pages 81 and 86 in "The First Relationship: Infant and Mother" by D. Stern, 1977; W. H. Freeman and Company, Figure 5.8 on page 79 from "A Primer of Infant Development" by T. G. R. Bower, Copyright © 1977; Harper & Row, Inc., an extract from page 25, "The Acquisition of Language: the Study of Developmental Psycholinguistics" by D. McNeill, 1970; Macmillan, London and Basingstoke, the extract from Beethoven's Heiligenstadt letter of 6th October 1802, from "Letters of Beethoven" by Emily Anderson; the MIT Press – an extract from page 222, "Language Development: Form and Function in Emerging Grammars" by Lois Bloom, 1970; extracts from pages 30 and 32, "Aspects of the Theory of Syntax" by N. Chomsky; an extract from pages 3, "Preliminaries to Speech Analysis" by R. Jakobson, C. G. M. Fant & M. Halle, 1952; Penguin Books Ltd. and Professor H. R. Schaffer, an extract from page 135 in "The Growth of Sociability" by H. R. Schaffer, 1971; Penguin Books Ltd., an extract from page 48 in "Maternal Deprivation Reassessed" in the Penguin Modern Psychology Series, ed. B. M. Foss, Copyright © Michael Rutter, 1972; Routledge & Kegan Paul Ltd., for extracts from pages 45, 74, 75, 93 and 96, in "Play, Dreams and Imitation" by J. Piaget, 1962; Spastics International Medical Publications and Dr. B. Touwen for Figure 12, page 43 and the related description on page 41 in "Neurological Development in Infancy" (Clinics in Developmental Medicine, No. 58) by B. Touwen, 1976; John Wiley and Sons Ltd. and Professor Adrian Fourcin for Figure 6, page 58 and an extract from page 68, "Acoustic Patterns and Speech Acquisition" by A. J. Fourcin in "The Development of Communication" edited by N. Waterson and C. Snow, 1978.

Contents

Glossary of Phonetic Symbols*

Fig. 4.1, age 22 hours

⟦ ⟧	double brackets enclosing vocant or closant sounds, the manner of production of these segmental sounds being in many (all?) instances innately determined: the actual sound value should be regarded as an approximation only to the usual value associated with the phonetic symbol, and inferences on place and manner of articulation based on adult articulatory phonetics are probably incorrect.
ə	the brief vowel sound of "th*e*" or "*a*lone"
h	as in "*h*allo" or "*h*elp"
x	an unidentificable click-like sound
( )	the enclosed sound is scarely heard
. or : or ::	increasing duration of a vowel or other continuous sound, e.g. a drawn-out "mm"

Fig. 4.3, age 2 days

ɣ	a sound like "g", but more frictional and drawn-out resulting in a throaty "ghh" quality
vp	an audible respiratory cycle, with very brief inspiratory and expiratory phases, used communicatively and referred to as a vocal pant
˜	indicates a nasal quality to the symbol beneath

Fig. 4.5, age 3 days

æ	the vowel sound in "h*a*t" or "c*a*t"
ŋ	a nasal sound heard mostly at the end*ing* of *Eng*lish words (though this latter is one of the few exceptions): it is very common as an initial sound in Bantu languages

Fig. 4.7, age 5 days

ʃ	"sh" as in "*sh*oe" (produced by the father soothing his child)

---

* Listed in chronological order of appearance in Chapters 4 and 8

Fig. 4.9, age 26 days

ʕ	is used here to represent an ingressive sound, produced on an indrawn breath, usually occurring at the end of the vocalisation; earlier examples have been labelled as such
ɛ	the vowel sound in "p*e*t" or "f*e*tch"

Fig. 4.10, age 1.6 months

g	as in "*g*o" or "do*g*"
ɑ	the vowel sound in "f*a*ther" or "p*a*rtner"

Fig. 4.11, age 3.5 months

a	somewhere between the vowel sound of "c*a*t" and "c*u*t" depending on which part of England one comes from
X	a somewhat guttural, frictional sound produced at the back of the tongue without laryngeal voicing, as in the Scottish "lo*ch*"
w	a sound frequently introduced between certain vo*w*el seq*u*ences as the lips are rounded

Fig. 4.12, age 4.5 months

ʀ	a light sustained palato-pharyngeal roughening or trill
au	as in "h*ow*"

Fig. 4.13, age 5.5 months

b	in "*b*a*b*y" or "*b*ye *b*ye"
β	a more continuous sound than "b" produced between the lips
u	the vowel sound in "wh*o*" or "sh*oe*"
ʊ	the vowel sound in "sh*ou*ld" or "p*u*t"

Fig. 4.17, age 7.6 months

eɪ	the diphthong in "p*ai*d" or "h*a*te" but here with the second vowel sound much less prominent
ɪ	the vowel sound of "*i*t"
o	there is no precise equivalent in English, perhaps the nearest being "N*o*vember" if it is pronounced more as written, rather than the usual /nəˈvɛmbə/

Fig. 4.18, age 8.5 months

d	as in "*d*a*dd*y"
ʔ	usually a sudden termination of a vowel sound or glottal stop, without a consonant being produced after, but here indicating the sudden onset of a vowel sound
t	in "*t*iny" or "pa*t*"
[ ]	single square brackets enclosing vowel-like or consonant-like sounds which are the immediate precursors of the segmental sounds occurring in spoken language: their manner of production is almost certainly identical to these but they are not yet being used linguistically

Fig. 4.20, age 9.4 months

j	this represents the initial sound of "*y*et" and bears no relation to the English "*j*ump" (which is /ʤ/)

Fig. 4.21, age 10.1 months

əu	the diphthong in "b*oa*t" or "sh*ow*"
ɒ	the vowel in "c*o*t" or "p*o*t"

Fig. 4.23, age 11.1 months

i	the vowel in "sh*e*" or "s*ee*"

Fig. 4.24, age 12.4 months

m	as in "*mumm*y"
/ /	oblique lines enclose the segmental sounds, vowels and consonants, of spoken language

Fig. 4.25, age 14.0 months

v	as in "*v*ery"
ɔ	the vowel sound in "*or*" or "th*ou*ght"
l	as in "*l*itt*le*"
ʌ	the vowel sound in "*u*p" or "j*u*mp"

Fig. 4.26, age 15.2 months

aɪ	the diphthong in "*I*" or "l*i*ght"
ʤ	as in "*j*ump" or "e*dge*"

Fig. 4.27, age 16.8 months

k	as in "*kick*" or "*c*limb"
z	as in "bee*s*" or "sea*s*"

Fig. 4.28, age 18.6 months

θ	as in "*th*ree" or "*th*ankyou"
p	as in "*p*ay" or "*p*lay"
k̬	a more voiced quality to "k" approaching "g"

Fig. 4.29, age 20.0 months

d̥	an unvoiced quality to "d" approaching "t"
ɪə	the diphthong in "d*ear*" or "h*ere*"

Fig. 8.2, Anna, age 8.4 months

ɸ	an unvoiced sound resembling "f" but made with the lips alone
ʉ	here somewhat as for /u/ with more pronounced rounding of the lips, as if about to whistle

Introduction

When does a young child first begin to talk? How is it that the cries which announce his arrival into the world change into the sounds, the words and sentences of our daily converse? Before developmental questions of this sort can be considered we need to have some notion of what happens when two normally accomplished speakers talk with one another. In the act of speaking words are produced and combined together into utterances which may be only one word, or may continue it seems interminably. In the process of joining words together a series of rules must be used according to the conventions of normal grammatical form. The particular words used and the choice of grammatical rules binding them together will convey something of what is in the speaker's mind. Before this can happen, the individual sounds of the words, the vowels and consonants, must be produced correctly within the different parts of the vocal tract. These phonemes must be arranged in an ordered sequence, a process which has its own special rules, and bound together in a rhythmic flow of syllables with the aid of subtle variations of tone, loudness, stress and voice quality. The nonverbal elements of speech are an essential component of the act of talking, and convey information which confirms, modifies or may even contradict what the speaker is saying.

The ideas, the wishes and feelings of the speaker are changed into the substance of words and tones which are then broadcast, as it were, into the surrounding air. In order to ensure that this flow of sound reaches its intended destination a number of rules bind speaker and listener so that attention is directed and meaning is derived from what is being said. Unlike the written word, when the reader's only options are to continue reading or close the book, the listener sooner or later changes his role and becomes in turn the speaker. There are a number of rules and devices by which the speaker signals she has finished and wishes to hand over her turn, or intends to retain it for a while longer. Similary the listener, by vocal interjections, facial expression or bodily movement signals with varying degrees of urgency his wish to take the turn over and speak. And as speaker and listener converse in this way, patterns of sound in the air convey meaning between the two, meaning which may be grounded in the immediate here and now of the objective world, or relate instead to the abstract meta-world of human ideas and feelings.

Language has so central a significance in the ordering of human affairs that it has come to exist in many people's minds in a dimension peculiarly its own, almost as if it were something apart from human nature. This independent existence is enhanced when one considers the written word. In this form language is astonishingly durable and we owe much of our knowledge of the past to inscriptions and documents dating back hundreds or thousands of years. So it is that the thoughts of philosophers and chroniclers, poets, soldiers and mystics continue to influence our present day attitudes and ideas. This seeming permanence of language, its potency in human intercourse, and its universality elevate it in the imagination to a metaphysical level where it can no longer be seen and talked about for what it is. Misconceptions abound, so deeply rooted in our culture that even those professionally involved in its study may be unaware of them.

Language is not a mystical thing-in-itself but is a direct product of our human nature, a necessary though mysterious consequence of the way the child perceives and communicates. In common with others, the view advanced here is that the development of language is intimately related to the social and cognitive development of the child, his grasp of interpersonal and objective reality. This, in its turn, is dependent on the well-ordered functioning of sensory, motor and other neurological processes which ensure efficient monitoring of the external world, and interaction with it. One has a recurring sense of amazement that children, relatively speaking so young in many accomplishments, are such adept performers in spoken language, and not only in language skills but in the varied processes through which people mutually adjust their interactions. The beginnings are to be found within a short time of birth, and what happens during the first two years or so is relevant to our theme.

Spoken language arises out of the way in which the child begins to make sense of the world about him and of his increasing understanding of the people in it. By the time the ground is adequately prepared for him to convey his thoughts verbally to others he has already acquired a remarkable level of skill in the control of the broadcasting medium, the vocal carrier wave, through which he will make his feelings and ideas heard. It is a long-standing personal view that the vocal behaviours of the first twelve to eighteen months of life are of fundamental importance to any adequate understanding of the development of spoken language yet they have been curiously devalued. An attempt is made to reveal something of the importance of these months through transcriptions of the utterances of individual children and their parents. Such transcriptions fail to convey the rhythms and harmonies of the utterances just as a musical score cannot convey to the reader all that it portrays unless it is heard. There are gains however. Vocal behaviours can be examined, dissected, timed, identified and related to context in a way which is impossible to the unaided ear. No-one need be deterred by the use of phonetic symbols if they are not already familiar with them; the sound-values to be attached to the symbols are soon acquired and are in any case approximations of decreasing accuracy with decreasing age.

If we are to understand something of the nature of language and the emergence of speech it is necessary to look first at other aspects of development in so far as these are relevant. Those well versed in a particular field will quickly detect a certain naivety, a too-elementary exploration of their field, and they must pass these sections by. It is necessary to provide a descriptive basis which steps over the boundaries between the major disciplines of psychology, linguistics and medicine. The second part of the book is concerned with the ways (it is premature to talk of causes) in which spoken language fails to develop normally. There is a great deal to learn about the normal from study of delayed or abnormal patterns of development of voice, speech and language. Similarly, for those whose work lies primarily in the clinical field, knowledge of the normal patterns of development and the processes which underlie them is essential. The cleft between the two, between the trained theorist and the experienced clinician, remains too sharp. Spoken language and human communication are complex, multifaceted activities, and the origins of disorder are mostly obscure. Our knowledge is as yet fragmentary and much remains to be learned. None of us may ignore the help afforded by a wide range of potential partners in alleviation of the suffering such disorders cause the children and their parents.

1 Attachment, Interaction and Communitive Behaviour

There is a natural tendency to divide our world into the world of people and their activities, and the inanimate, physical world. If we are to understand the nature of spoken language and its early development it is essential to look both at infant behaviour in relation to other human beings, and at the way in which children begin to make sense of the physical characteristics of their surroundings. The origins of language are embedded in these activities.

Though it seems natural and appropriate to us to make this two-fold division of the environment, it is probably less meaningful to the infant who is in the first stages of exploration of the world he has recently entered. The skills he needs to perceive and to make sense of his mother, his identification of her as a person and the meanings he can extract from her various activities are little different from those by which he acquires an understanding of the objects which surround him, and of their arrangements in space and time. It is convenient to preserve the distinction so long as it is realized that orderly development in either is dependent on increasing skill in the other.

It is a biological necessity that the newborn infant is cared for and protected, kept warm, fed and clean, and free from infection. In the human child this process continues in various suitably modified forms for many years until he is able to fend for himself, meaning that he is competent to ensure an adequate level of selfcare and that he can order his own life. This is usually termed being independent, but independence is a state which cannot be achieved even in the adult without numerous provisos being made which greatly dilute the concept. Human behaviour is characterized by social interaction, the formation of attachments of various degrees of intensity and of interdependence at a variety of levels. It is hardly to be wondered that such typically human behaviours are at the root of the process of bonding between the mother and her child. Their origins are not human at all but can be studied in mammalian and phylogenetically earlier forms of animal behaviour, particularly amongst the more gregarious species. Such ethological studies have contributed much to the understanding of human behaviour, and serve to remind one of the astonishing longevity of bonding behaviour and of the complexity of interaction between individuals in non-human species.

It is one thing to assert the necessity of certain behaviour patterns which will ensure the survival of the newborn until he and she are able in turn to care for their own young, and so secure the future of the race. It is quite another matter to achieve a reasonable understanding of the various processes by which parents and child not only secure his physical survival, but ensure that he will grow up with a full repertoire of social and cognitive skills.

The Neonatal Period

A number of factors have been described, operating between the mother and her child, which develop and strenghten the bond of attachment from the moment of birth.

Mother to Child

A mother who is given her new born infant will either hold him or if unable to, will have him lying as close to her as possible where she can see him. Characteristically, she will gaze intently, will talk to him and about him with those around, and will begin gently to touch and explore him. It has been found that there is a definite pattern of touching which develops over the next few hours and days. Touching begins very gently, with her fingertips directed towards his hands and feet and face, and this changes to a more encompassing caress directed to his trunk and body as a whole, using a grip which involves the palms of the hands (Rubin, 1963; Klaus, Kennell, Plumb, and Zuehlke, 1970). She tends to pitch her voice higher than the level she uses in ordinary conversation and in general it appears that the new born is more responsive to the female than the male voice. It may be that this is due in part to the effects of a physiological middle ear deafness, due to the presence of fluid in the middle ear clefts until it has drained away. The effect would be to impair hearing more for lower frequency sounds.

Improbable though it might be, especially to those who consider the infant to be a passive recipient of stimuli with no ability to select or process what is going on around him, the newborn is able to respond actively to an adult speaker. Condon and Sander (1974) studied videotape recordings of infants from twelve hours to two days old and by scrutinizing the film at one twentieth of a second intervals and less, were able to demonstrate that movements occurred of the fingers, the hands and arms, and of the baby's head and feet which were synchronous in time with certain features of the speech. This synchrony was often sustained by an infant across long sequences of words, and has led to the conclusion that "the neonate participates immediately and deeply in communication and is not an isolate which slowly develops such skills after many months" (Condon, 1974). This behaviour has been called entrainment or interactional synchrony.

There is a ground swell of rhythmical activity which the mother takes advantage of to interact with her child. The patterns of sleeping, feeding and wakefulness are progressively recognized by her so that she is able to adjust her activities and be with him during his alert periods, when effective interaction can take place.

In addition to these behavioural interactions, there are other more physical and biochemical ways by which the mother affects her child and develops the bond between them. The warmth of her body; the aggregate of organic substances which contributes to her particular smell and which facilitates the infant's recognition of her; the transfer of cellular and other material during breast feeding serve to strengthen the attachment.

Child to Mother

Until relatively recently there has been a strong tendency to think that the attachment taking place between mother and child was one-sided, that it was the effect of the mother on her child that mattered. This was if anything increased by the concept of imprinting introduced by Lorenz (1952, 1969) in his studies of geese, though through no fault of his. Imprinting has come to be thought of as a virtually automatic process, with the young irrestibly and permanently effected by the first sight of the mother. The fault may be due in part to the word itself, bearing the suggestion of a once-for-all photographic process. Animal behavioural studies have shown that the phenomenon owes a great deal to learning. It develops maximally in birds some time after birth, and the intensity of imprinting is related to the amount of effort exerted by the young in their efforts to follow the "mother" object. It is clearly necessary to avoid too facile a use of the concept in considering the nature of attachment, and of the notion of "critical period" with which it is associated. Imprinting can only take place within certain time limits and these are therefore critical for its appearance. The term originates from study of the complex cellular changes taking place in embryological development, referring to the times when non-differentiated tissue may or may not develop into say, differentiated neural tissue with no possibility of further change. The term has been appropriated from cellular biology and applied to various psychological phenomena of a developmental nature, particularly in attempts to explain disordered behaviour or the failure of certain skills or behaviours to develop.

If we consider the effect a baby has on those around, it is quickly apparent that the interaction is far from being a unilateral mother to infant process. People of both sexes behave in a very similar fashion when confronted by a baby, making due allowance for the inhibition or lack of it in the behaviour directed towards him. They adopt a different posture, the facial displays, the language (not that it can always be called that), the voice and its prosodic characteristics, are all quite different from those used in ordinary interaction. They may end by touching, caressing and picking up to fondle or kiss. This is not restricted to adults, but may also be seen in children, often quite young, and more readily in girls. The universal nature of this reaction suggests that it is innate and is a specific response to some feature or constellation of features in the infant. The reaction is not confined to human infants but may be elicited by the young of most species of mammals, and by birds. It is probably relevant to add that these are animals in whom a strong attachment between parents and infant is essential if the young are to survive. The characteristics of "babyishness" are familiar to all and scarcely need further elaboration. Tinbergen (1951) explains the adult babying response by saying that the features of the infant act as stimuli which release parental reaction.

It is necessary to think of the process of attachment not as a mother to child movement, nor as the simple, reflex operation of instinctive behaviour released by certain facial and other characteristics, but as a complex pattern of interaction. The concepts of attachment and mother-child interaction cannot be thought of as two psychologically different processes. Rather, the two are bound together in a tight spiral, a double helix of mutuality, in which interaction leads to attachment which leads to interaction at a higher—or deeper—level, which leads to the formation of a stronger bond of attachment, and so on.

The visual system of the human infant is well developed at birth, and this competence will be further examined later. Desmond, Rudolph, and Phitaksphraiwan (1966) have demonstrated that the newly born can see, that he has visual preferences, that he will respond to sound and this state of quiet alertness may last for almost the whole of the first hour after birth. In a compelling phrase, Klaus and Kennell (1976) conclude that "for one hour after birth he (the infant) is ideally equipped for the important first meeting with his parents", see Fig. 1.1. In the early hours and days after birth, the ability of the child to see and to gaze at his mother releases or awakens intense emotional forces in her, and in the father and others who might of necessity be involved in the caretaking process. The infant becomes human, becomes a person, and this eye-to-eye contact is supremely important to the mother.

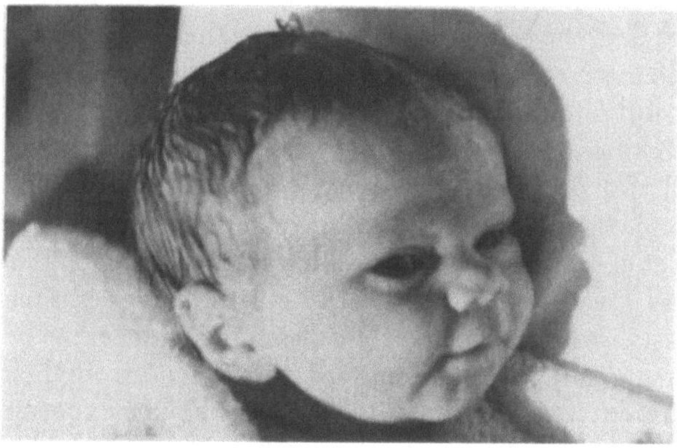

Fig. 1.1. Alert, wide-eyed appearance of girl 30 minutes after birth. (Courtesy of Dr. David Kemp)

The infant's cry is a source of interaction which it is difficult to ignore, urging the mother to his side to determine the cause and leading her to pacify and comfort him or to start feeding. The characteristics of the normal cry are discussed in more detail in chapter 4.

It has already been noted that the child, from soon after birth, will respond to the voice and movements of adults as they talk to him. This interactional synchrony must also be regarded as a two-way process, and not merely the effect of the adult on the child. It will be quickly appreciated by any who read the descriptions of the work carried out by Condon and Sanders that it took hours of detailed and exhaustive study to detect the responses of the infant. They were analyzing frame by frame film which had been taken at 24 and 48 frames per second. One might be tempted to ask how relevant such a behaviour is, if it is so difficult to demonstrate. The answer must be that the ordinary observer does not detect all, or perhaps many of the details of the patterns of movement by which the infant responds. The overall effect, or gestalt, is however very real and immediately marks the baby as being vital, responsive and alert, in contrast with the one who lies passive and still for whatever reason.

There are other factors which operate from the first hours after birth, related more to the effects which the infant has on his mother's awareness of her role. The sight of the new-born usually arouses intense feelings of wonder (and of relief), of a sense of his fragility and total physical dependence on her. Helplessness is itself a powerful releaser of caring behaviour, evidence of which is present all around us in the activities of individuals and of human organizations in many subtle and covert forms. It comes into prominence in times of earthquake, flood, accident and other calamities. Helplessness on the one's part, and responsibility for his arrival and for his care on the other's combine with the factors already mentioned to establish a bond of attachment between mother and child with remarkable speed in the early postnatal period.

It is doubtful that this is the full story. From the moment she knows that she is pregnant the mother, with varying degrees of conscious awareness, has been preparing herself for the time when her child is born. It would not be unreasonable to suggest that the process starts before conception takes place in the majority of pregnancies, in the desire and intention to have a child. The beginnings of attachment can then be traced back in the human to a time before there was any infant with whom the mother could interact, before she became aware of his movements in utero and before the physical and hormonal changes she experiences as a direct result of pregnancy. Attachment is not only a phenomenon associated with the sight and sound and smell of the baby, of his activity and his dependence, but is grounded in the emotional and cognitive processes of the parents. That this is so may be seen in the reactions of grief and ensuing depression which a mother feels when her child is stillborn. She has already formed an attachment and her grief is real and appropriate. This contrasts with the apparently callous and indifferent behaviour of the medical and nursing staff of the labour ward, which stems from their inability to develop any attachment to the dead foetus, denied as they are exposure to the features which elicit attachment behaviours after birth, and in which they can normally share for a short time.

Early Opportunities for Interaction

As the neonate develops, the most obvious changes in the way in which he relates to those around him concern the use of vision. From early on he turns towards the light and stares persistently at the brighter illuminated area formed by the window. The human face holds a particular fascination and he watches his mother's face with increasing intensity, see Fig. 1.2.

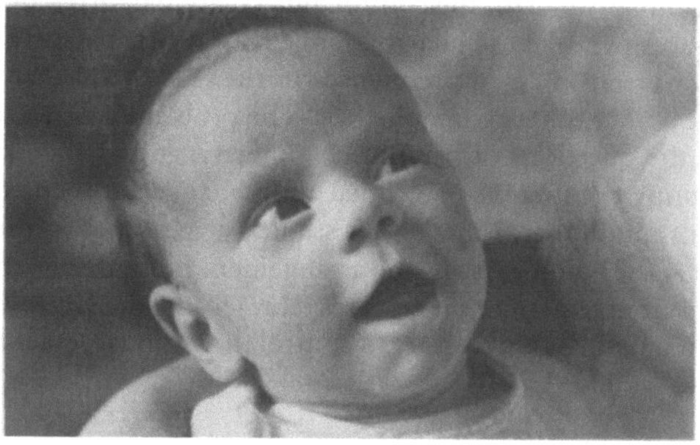

Fig. 1.2. Interaction with mother, whilst held in her arm; same girl as in Fig. 1.1, now aged 4 weeks. (Courtesy of Dr. David Kemp)

In the early weeks much of his time is spent asleep, but when awake he is involved in a variety of activities with his mother. The basic routines of feeding, nappy changing, bathing and changing clothes necessitate a good deal of interaction. The daily pattern of events itself helps him to begin to order his world and by the end of the first month he is already beginning to show an incipient awareness of these routines. More important for the development of social skills is the recurring opportunity to interact with his mother. During a feed for instance he will stop sucking and gaze intently at his mother, who if she is not already watching him, becomes aware of the change in his activity and gazes at him. Mother and child may look at each other in this mutual regard for some time, perhaps thirty seconds or more, until one or other changes the situation either to continue feeding or to play. At this age the infant's focal length is about 8 inches, a typical distance between the two faces in feeding, and there are endlessly repeated opportunities for the child to register, to assimilate and recognize his mother's face, and subsequently to learn the variety of expressions which she uses to initiate and regulate episodes of playful interaction.

The Infant's Recognition of the Face

First comes the need to recognize the human face. From the way in which the infant responds so selectively to his mother's face and to those adults who come frequently into his world, it would be reasonable to assume that he is born with the ability to do so. This is true, but in a special and initially limited way; recognition of the human face shows a clearly defined developmental progression. Fantz (1961) used the infant's duration of gaze as an indicator of the preference for a particular visual display, inferring that if the infant looks longer at one display or picture rather than another, he is indicating a preference for it. His experiment involved the use of three pictures, each the approximate shape and size of a human head, in which one was a simple representation of the face in black on a pink background, the next showed the same features but arranged randomly, and the third, control display simply had the upper part of the shape blacked in. There was a clear preference for the "face" in comparison with the control, but a marginal difference in visual fixation for the "face" over the irregularly arranged facial elements. He submitted that there was a consistent if small preference for the "face" and that there is an unlearned innate ability to recognize the face. The problem is however not so easily resolved, and the questions of stimulus complexity, and of the most appropriate ways of measuring the infant's perceptual ability have led others to conclude that this view needs modifying. Fantz's later studies suggest that in the one-week-old child or less it is the complexity of the arrangement presented to the infant rather than the actual arrangement of the features representing the face which engages the attention (Fantz, 1965). It is necessary to control the various elements of the overall

Simple dots or angles.		Under 6 weeks
Eye section alone; under portion of face unnecessary.		10 weeks
Eye section still suffices, but under half of face must be present even though mouth movements only fleetingly noticed; motion facilitates.	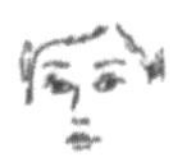	12 weeks
Eye section still suffices, with wide individual differences. Mouth gradually noticed, its movements particularly effective. Wide mouth best. Plastic model of adult effective.	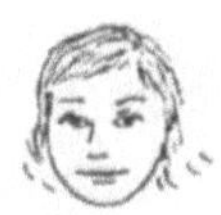	20 weeks
Effectiveness of eyes lessens; mouth movements generally necessary, especially widely drawn mouth. Still no differentiation of individual faces.	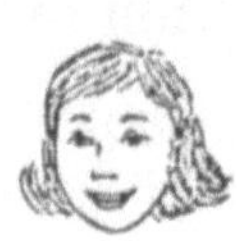	24 weeks
Attention to face as such lessens; recognition of facial expression begins, with interest in other children. Progressive differentiation of individual faces.	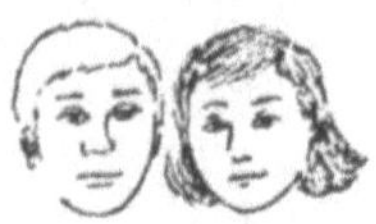	30 weeks

Fig. 1.3. The stimuli necessary to elicit a smile at various ages (from Bower, T. G. R. [1977]: A Primer of Infant Development; by permission W. H. Freeman and Company, San Francisco)

display, and if this is done carefully it is found that the infant prefers particular elements, such as dots, which with increasing age need to be displayed with other elements in order to gain a response (Haaf and Bell, 1967). Initially then it is certain visual features to which the young infant responds preferentially, rather than the face as such. In any other than experimental conditions, the most likely source of such features for the infant is the human face itself. The shift in importance from specific facial features such as the high contrast afforded between the white sclera of the eye and the iris, or between the inner canthus of the eyelids and the sclera, to the face as a whole, begins to take place during the first three months and becomes established not long thereafter. The trend is almost certainly related to the infant's increasing cognitive skills, shown by the control of attention and the amount of information which can be processed. It is too much for the infant of six weeks to scan the whole face and his attention is directed probably through innate mechanisms to the most characteristic and salient features. The way in which facial perception develops is usefully and clearly summarized in Fig. 1.3 using the smile as an indicator of recognition.

The Smile

Smiling is one of the behaviours of considerable importance in the formation of attachments between the infant and his parents, and has attracted a great deal of interest and study. Numerous arguments arise over whether a particular facial expression is a smile or due to wind in the stomach. Something approaching a smile can be seen on the face of young infants when asleep, or if awake, not in relation to a specific stimulus such as his mother's gaze or playful interaction. It is on the contrary vague, lacking the characteristics of a real smile, and occurring inappropriately, incidental to the activites going on around. By the time the infant is about three weeks old the smile becomes more convincing and seems to be more related to people, so that his mother's voice is quite likely to bring it on. At six weeks old the smile is unequivocal, quite different from the innate "smile" of the neonate, and most readily elicited by the human face. That the infant of this age is not responding specifically to the face but to certain salient features has been noted above, and the smile has proved to be a useful indicator of the child's perception of the face. The stages in the development of the smile have been attributed to a combination both of genetic factors, which determine the neuromotor pathways from the brain to the muscles of facial expression, and by the processes of growth. This conclusion of Bower (1977) is based on the findings of studies carried out on children born after varying periods of intrauterine life. Infants normally start to smile at the human face at six weeks, representing a conceptual age of forty six weeks. It is the conceptual age which is significant, so that whether the infant was some weeks premature, or was late in arriving, the smile nevertheless appears at about forty six weeks from conception.

The smile is highly rewarding to an infant's parents, forming with the intent, face to face gaze a compelling mechanism for further strengthening the bonds of attachment. Within a few weeks of its appearance it is put to good use by the infant, who can by now control it sufficiently to turn it on in order to achieve some goal, such as the renewal of interest and interaction on the part of his mother. Though smiling has so far been considered in an entirely social context, recent work suggests the likelihood that there are other reasons for the infant to break into a smile, and this aspect will be examined further under the child's cognitive abilities (p. 43). Certainly it would be wrong to imagine there is only one smile. On the contrary, as Bower states (1977, p. 47), "smiles may be qualitatively different in the infant for qualitatively different situations". Laughter has aroused less interest and its study has been relatively neglected. It appears to have a different origin from smiling, and follows a different developmental course. It is not present at birth, in contrast with the cry which proclaims the newborn infant's capacity for physical existence separate from his mother, and which is such a prominent feature of the early weeks of life. Laughter is first heard at about four months, usually as a result of tickling and other direct and often quite vigorous stimulation. During the previous month the infant has been able to show his pleasure at such friendly handling by smiling, cooing and various forms of excited behaviour involving the pattern of breathing and movements of the arms and legs. Somewhat later Sroufe and Waters (1976) state that auditory stimuli become more effective in inducing laughter, and by ten to twelve months this has in its turn been replaced by visual events, with a strong tendency towards the more subtle and cognitive type of stimulation, involving the creation of expectancy and the sudden release of tension during play.

Patterns of Interaction

Smiling and laughter, the tense, worried face of displeasure or anxiety, crying and the various types of vocal behaviour all have a part to play in communication. They are in fact the more immediately obvious components of an immensely intricate and subtle signalling system which develops between the infant and his mother, his father and siblings, and others involved intimately in his care. The patterns of interaction between mother and child have been studied in considerable detail by Stern and his associates (Stern, 1974, 1977). They have contributed greatly to an understanding of the ways in which interaction is initiated, continued or adjusted, and brought to an end, and the parts played by mother and child in regulating the flow of their joint activity.

Mutual Gaze

The earliest interaction is probably the mutual gaze, made possible when the infant is held in the *en face* position and which most easily takes place during feeding. At about six weeks the quality of eye-to-eye contact changes because the infant becomes more capable of holding his mother's eyes and shows an increased intensity of expression with widening and brightening of the eyes. This change may be partly instrumental in deepening the level of attachment in association with the true, social smile. The effect on the mother is to increase the level of social interaction.

The relationship has been essentially one-sided up to this point, but from now on the mother can discern the active, sharing nature of her infant's activities. The subliminal synchrony of interaction described by Condon and Sanders, which doubtless conveys the subconscious assurance of a living and responsive child, is overshadowed by the clear manifestation of active participation in their relationship.

Modulation of Interaction

An episode of interaction may be initiated at almost any time when the infant is awake and alert. A pause in the rhythmical sucking during a feed may result in the sharing of gaze; after the appropriate moment of pause the mother may encourage her child to continue feeding. It may happen that a little interlude of play takes place instead, because of some slight change in the activity or facial expression of her child. She may start talking and combine this with a gentle joggling motion of her arms, or tickle him; she may smilingly turn her face away and suddenly turn back to him with a "bo" and repeat this several times, until he no longer coos pleasurably and looks expectant, but instead begins to tire and loses interest. His mother can then decide either to stop the game or to change one or other element of her play—physical activity, head movement, facial expression, vocalization, or the timing of these different components in order to reawaken his interest and his level of arousal and attention.

This type of interaction is a highly dynamic process, sensitively adjusted during the course of the play episode, with further adjustments occurring between one episode and the next, until that particular play session is over. The controlling and adjusting mechanisms which are brought into action include those features of interpersonal behaviour familiar to everyone from consideration of adult non-verbal modes of communication, and of the numerous facial, bodily, positional and other changes which accompany speech. The importance of the work of Stern and his colleagues is to show what every parent of a young child unconsciously assumes—that the interaction taking place between them and their child shares the basic characteristics of adult interaction. Unless completely new, categorically different behaviours are to be brought into play as a concomitant of the child's birth it is difficult to see how it could be otherwise.

Facial Expressions and Their Part in Interaction

Facial expression plays an important part, so that the more sophisticated forms of interaction cannot begin until the infant's neurology is sufficiently mature, and his cognitive abilities sufficiently developed to permit an adequate span of attention; and for him to perceive, register and process particular configurations of facial appearance, and their alteration. Stern (1977) selects five basic expressions as being typical of the mother's repertoire. There is the neutral, essentially expressionless face, the smile and the frown which need no further description. In addition there are two which he labels the "mock-surprise" and the "oh, you poor dear" expressions. The former is characterized by wide open eyes, elevated eyebrows and a widely open mouth, and at the same time the head is raised and slightly up-tilted. There are variations on this theme depending on the degree of completeness of the display, on the amount of smile incorporated, and on the movement and position of the head and face in relation to the child. The "poor dear" expression combines elements of the frown with this expression resulting in slightly knit eyebrows but with the eyes opened wide rather than narrowed, and the mouth open rather than pursed.

Facial expressions are used differently from the normal way with adults and older children. They are developed more slowly, are exaggerated in the extent of their display, and in the time for which they are held. This restricted range permits the infant to identify much more quickly than he otherwise would the basic set of expressions and to associate them with various phases and states of interaction. Once this has been done numerous variations can be introduced in which individual basic motor units of facial expression such as lip spreading, tensing, parting, or pouting can be combined with other features affecting the eyes, the forehead and brows, the nose, and cheeks, the posture and tilt of the head, to provide a richly varied source of information. Certain positions and movements of facial features, initially restricted in their range of combination, are used purposefully to signal to the infant various aspects of the course and progress of an interaction episode.

An episode may well be initiated by the mock-surprise expression, signalling the mother's readiness to become involved, and stimulating the infant to do so. Her smile signals the continuation, and the pleasure associated with the episode, whilst if the interaction is not going well she may signal her concern with the "poor dear" face, changing the pattern of the interaction in some way in order to maintain it. A pause can be introduced or the episode brought to an end by turning her eyes and head slightly away, averting her gaze and frowning slightly. The blank, neutral face is clearly no invitation for the infant to embark on an interactive episode, especially if his mother's head and face are turned away. It needs to be remembered however that the infant is not simply a receiver of signals, complying with the information conveyed to him about his mother's state of mind and intentions. He may well be active in initiating the play, and in obliging his mother to continue despite her signals to the contrary. How successful he is will of course depend on many other factors over which he can have no control.

These episodes and sequences of interaction can take place many times during the day, during all the various procedures devoted to his individual care. Even if the episodes of play are restricted to these times of unavoidable personal contact between the child and his caretakers there are innumerable opportunities for him to learn the basic routines of interaction. In many families it is possible to provide a great deal more, as his periods of wakefulness lengthen, purely for the joy the mother can experience in being with her child, with no demands made on either of them other than to delight in each other's company.

Interaction and Emotional Development

Playful interaction has no predetermined goal to be achieved and this frees both participants from any constraints of obligation, enabling each to explore the other's actions and reactions, and so increase the depth of attachment between them. In the course of their interaction the mother will endeavour to gain and to hold her child's attention by adjusting carefully the level of stimulation. His state of arousal will inevitably swing between excitement and boredom, between increasing and lessening degrees of interest, and his mother will modulate her behaviour accordingly. She can do this by altering the nature of the game she is playing with him, changing from a more specifically visual game to one in which the voice or physical activity predominate. The nature of these games can be changed endlessly, and so can the various combinations of vocal, visual and physical play. A pattern of interaction is set up in which a particular play is repeated several times, but the details are progressively changed and novel features introduced before the child becomes habituated, and loses interest. If the infant is denied these well-controlled signalling procedures by which his level of arousal can be adjusted or is unable to detect them, he swings violently in one direction or the other, becoming overexcited or irritable and unhappy. Once either extreme has been reached the infant is unable to respond and communication is at an end. The most skilfull of parents will not be able to avoid these more extreme swings at times, but there may be occasions when they actively encourage the less violent alterations of attention and mood. It seems that child and parent can benefit from this crossing of the boundaries above and below an optimum range of arousal. To quote Stern (1977, p. 86) "... only when a boundary is exceeded is the infant forced to execute some coping or adaptive manoeuvre to correct or avoid the situation or to signal to the mother to alter the immediate stimulus environment. The infant behaviours, like any others, require constant practice, constant opportunities under slightly different conditions to become fully developed adaptive behaviours. Second, unless the mother frequently risks exceeding a boundary, whether by design or miscalculation, she will be unable to help stretch and expand the infant's growing range of tolerance for stimulation."

The tempo of the pattern of interaction is as important a means of modulating the infant's behaviour and arousal as the nature of the stimulus itself. This applies not only to the timing of activities within an episode of interaction but to the pauses between episodes as the mother and child settle down briefly in a moment of respite before the next. The mother is able to introduce variation by altering the rate at which she conducts a particular game or series of play episodes, speeding up or slowing down more and more, with her infant on the tenterhooks of anticipation waiting for the climax and resolution of the episode.

Careful judgement is required in all this in order to maintain his interest without making him fearful or unduly excited. The infant signals his state by the same sort of devices that are used by his mother. Smiling, eager anticipation, cooing and laughter, contortions of the limbs and body, the position of the head and face all indicate that he is keenly alert and willing her to continue. This may change after some unduly boisterous or sudden, unexpected activity, or the use of an overloud voice on her part, the smile then being replaced by a sober, wary expression. This may be accompanied by a change of gaze, taking his eyes off his mother, but retaining her in his peripheral vision, waiting to see what she will do next. These are signals for her to restructure her play, reducing the tension and anxiety to a level which he can more easily accept. In the more extreme instance, the sober, wary face turns into a grimace, with agitated whimpers soon to be followed by frank crying if suitable counter-action is not quickly instituted.

The Elaboration of a Communication System

By the time the infant is six months old he will have mastered the basic signals which regulate the ebb and flow of interaction, and with his mother will have developed an intricate system of communication. The signals used, their sequential ordering and the timing of their appearance become organized almost into units of play activity, which are arranged into broader and more loosely knit patterns. It is as if a syntax of play behaviour is being evolved, with guidelines being laid down for when to take turns, when to make a response, when to act in unison participating in the same routine at the same time, when to hold back and wait for what is coming next. It cannot be doubted that the fundamental conventions which govern the behaviours of the adult speaker and listener participating in a conversation are laid down long before a single word can be uttered. Individuals vary greatly in their ability to provide this sort of ordered but flexible and attention-holding stimulation. Some have very limited play routines, more usually seen in fathers especially if they do not receive the necessary encouragement to play from an early age with their children. Some parents seem to have very little sensitivity in detecting the points in time at which to change the nature or tempo of their play. Some, either because of reasons originating in their own upbringing or because of their particular personality and attitudes, seem unable to derive any pleasure from this sort of playful interaction. A great deal more, painstaking enquiry is required before pronouncements can be made on the effects which such parental behaviours will have on the formation of attachment and subsequent emotional development, the attainment of social skills, and the acquisition and use of spoken language by the child.

Awareness of Strangers

Soon after the end of the first six months a major change in the infant's attitude to people begins to appear. At six months he is friendly towards strangers but a month later is showing definite reserve towards them. A month or two further on he may become fearful in their presence, clinging desperately to someone he knows, turning his face away and burying it in the shoulder of the person carrying him, with all the signs and sounds of distress. It is often thought that the appearance of stranger fear comes suddenly and is fully developed, as if a stepwise change both in emotional maturation and interpersonal relationships had taken place. The available evidence does not support this. At six months the infant will occasionally show shyness, or even slight anxiety when the non-familiar person approaches rather too near or too quickly (Sheridan, 1975). In his studies of the development of the smiling response, Ambrose (1961) noted that at about fourteen weeks infants would stare rather than smile at strangers, or that there was a definite latency period before the smile appeared. A real developmental shift does occur, but it seems likely that it is not necessarily the stranger as such, but his or her behaviour which arouses distress. The infant is more likely to display concern if the non-familiar person approaches too vigorously, bearing down rapidly and talking loudly as she does so. Personal space is important to the young child, in the way that it is to the adult, but is frequently abused, and many people behave as if their greeting must take the form of physical contact. For his part the child is forced into close proximity with someone with whom he has no communication system, and who almost certainly uses a set of visual and other signals which are quite different from those developed over the previous months in his home. The more probable the interaction the more likely is the infant to show distress, and to become frankly fearful. The effect of a strange place may be such that the infant in the absence of his mother, will approach a stranger, whereas if his mother is near and a stranger approaches, he may show signs of extreme fear. Haith and Campos (1977) conclude that stranger distress is neither as predictable nor as universal at any one age as once thought. In support of this is a personal clinical observation that it is exceptional to see the phenomenon in children of seven or eight months and older who are brought by their parents into a strange building and a strange clinic room, and confronted by strange adults in order to have their hearing tested. On the contrary, many of these infants actively solicit the interest and attention of the medical and other staff, taking the initiative in starting an interaction as they sit on their mother's lap.

Separation and the Objects of Attachment

Closely associated with the infant's potential anxiety in the presence of strangers, and coming a little later in time is the anxiety which quickly becomes manifest when the infant is separated from his mother. Tears and other forms of protest can be seen long before this age, but the protest is over the fact of separation and not separation specifically from mother. In the early months the reaction is virtually indiscriminate but from eight months or so, the distress of separation relates to his mother alone, or to a very restricted group of people. Schaffer and Emerson (1964) found that the majority of children in their study formed their initial attachment to one person, but 29% had already developed multiple attachments from the first time a specific attachment could be demonstrated. Three months later, only 41% of the children had one "attachment object" (their term for the person to whom the child is showing attachment behaviour), and by eighteen months old this figure had decreased to 13%. As far as the individual people are concerned, they found that attachment objects are generally arranged in a hierarchy with the principal object being the mother. With increasing age there was an increasing tendency for others, and in particular the father, to take on this position, so that by eighteen months nearly a third directed their most intense attachment behaviour at some individual other than the mother.

The finding that people other than the mother can be the object of the child's attachment raises the question of the nature of the child's experience leading up to and determining attachment. A prevailing and essentially mechanistic view was that attachment or as it was then usually termed, dependence, would naturally take place to the one who was responsible for his feeding and physical care. Schaffer (1971) concluded otherwise:

"Instead, the characteristics that determined most clearly the choice of object were, in the first place, the individual's responsiveness to the infant's signals for attention, and, in the second place, the amount of interaction which the adult spontaneously initiated with the infant. The amount of time spent together (at least above a certain level) appeared to play little part. In as many as 39 per cent of infants the principal object at eighteen months of age was someone other than the most available individual—generally the father, despite his absence for all but a brief part of the day." (p. 135)

The effect of these observations has been twofold. It has stimulated interest in an area of research which up until then had been virtually ignored. There can be no doubt that the father has an important place in encouraging cognitive and emotional development in the child, and with present day changes in the attitudes of the parents towards employment and domesticity, the father's participation will be even more important. The other effect is a frank acknowledgement that the infant is much more than something to be fed, kept clean and warm, and otherwise left in his carrycot to stare at nothing more stimulating than the kitchen ceiling. This is reflected in the great increase in interest in the infant as a worthwhile and legitimate object of scientific enquiry, and an almost astonished awareness that the very young child has a remarkable range of cognitive and communicative skills.

Communitive Behaviour

In considering the underlying nature of separation anxiety it seems likely that the child is not, after all, concerned about the departure of the person who is his primary source of food and comfort. It is almost certainly, as Bower (1977) affirms, the departure of the one with whom he is best able to communicate, and who may have been replaced by someone who does not have any idea of his particular communication system, that creates the anxiety. Of course, in the majority of young children, the one who provides the basic care, and the one who is his most adept communication partner, are one and the same. The corollary of Bower's thesis is that separation anxiety should diminish as the child becomes more skilled in communication with those around, and he notes a clear association between the child's increasing mastery of language and the progressive decline of separation anxiety, starting sometime before the second birthday.

Words entrain our thinking rather more than we might be prepared to admit and it is interesting that "attachment" has largely replaced "dependence". Bowlby (1958) wished to emphasize the differences between physical and emotional dependence, and "attachment" was considered to be a more accurate and less charged term for the underlying concept. Since then the crucial importance of communication has been recognized in virtually all aspects of human society and its organization, in the mass and for the individual. A prevailing characteristic of humankind is seen to be that of communication, and there can be no argument with this. The proliferation of the printed, broadcast and televised forms of verbal communication are sufficient evidence, and this is paralleled by the increased interest in the scientific study of language and of human communication processes. But is this recent understanding sufficiently comprehensive? Does the term "communication" reach sufficiently into the core of our human nature? Probably not. Human beings are certainly communicating animals, but before this they are social animals, in whom the sense of "being with" one another is so deeply ingrained, so fundamental a feature that it is unremarkable, so universal that it is not worth mentioning. But we cannot assume that this is the case for the young child, other than as he brings the tendency into the world with him in his genetic make-up.

Before considering the importance of this concept of "being with", or what might be called communion or communitive behaviour, in the development of the child, it may be helpful to digress briefly into the world of the adult. It is difficult to identify any non-trivial human activity which does not involve other human beings. There are many solitary occupations, the process of writing being one that comes immediately to mind, but none has any significance outside a social, interpersonal context. The matter goes deeper than this. The necessity to earn a living may drive certain individuals into isolated work situations but a more predominant characteristic of work is that it necessitates the direct and complex interaction of many individuals. If one examines what people choose to do, rather than what they are obliged to do, the picture does not change. Mealtimes, especially at work, could provide the opportunity to be alone, but the tendency is to seek the company of others rather than the reverse. Many forms of leisure involve joint activity, and pictures of crowded holiday beaches and beauty spots suggest that the company of others, being with and amongst others, is an essential element. Those who decry such crowded places might ask themselves why they choose to attend conferences, lectures, sporting events, concerts and theatres, when the same end could ostensibly be achieved by reading the written reports, listening to recordings or watching television. It is the extra dimension that is added by being present, being with the audience and with the speaker or the players, which makes the essential difference.

Interrelation in Activity

This sense of shared activity is best described by the word "communion" defined as "an action or situation involving sharing in common, ... an interrelation in activity" (Webster, 1971). Communion, or the active form "communitive behaviour" may be expressed in the more general ways outlined above, or in the more intense, closely knit relationships involved in friendship, in marriage and within the family. The principle which underlies attachment is not one of adhesion or interlocking, but of the working out of the desire, indeed the necessity, to be with another. Evidence for the intuitive grasp of this concept can be found in the writings of several people. Stern (1977) uses the phrase "be with" three times on one page (p. 81):

"The immediate goal of a face-to-face play interaction is to have fun, to interest and delight and *be with* one another ... We are dealing with a human happening, conducted solely with interpersonal 'moves', with no other end in mind than to *be with* and enjoy someone else." And especially (my italics again) *"The infant first has to learn to be with someone* and to create and share the experiences that a relationship is built on."

Bower (1977) makes the same point by implication when he writes "It seems to me very unlikely that babies can tolerate solitude either. When their mothers go off and leave them they are, for all intents and purposes, alone, completely isolated, because they have learned to communicate and interact with one specific person." And he uses the word itself:

"This behaviour is intrinsically social; it is a distinctively social behaviour. Interactional synchrony was not elicited by any of the sounds used in this experiment except human speech. This kind of communication—*or communion*—is obviously of great importance in a mother's feeling that her baby is responding to her." (p. 32, my italics)

The negative aspect of fear of being alone is combined and worked out in the child with the positive necessity to be at one with other similar beings. The extent to which this is achieved is always a relative matter, rarely if ever fully worked out between one another in life as we presently know and understand it. And just as adult life shows a hierarchy of depth of attachment and of degree of interdependence in any one individual's extraordinarily far ranging set of friends, colleagues and acquaintances, so the infant from the time that attachment is first demonstrable shows the same ordering of relationships with those around him. It would be utopian, or perhaps more aptly, a heavenly ideal for all humans to be at one with one another. In the world as we know it, it is essential for the child to acquire quickly the ability to discriminate between those with whom he is secure and those who might be a hazard to him. It is always a matter of concern to see children who for a variety of reasons, whether arising in the home, or through developmental delay or because of mental handicap, show no ability to discriminate friend, and sometimes even parent, from stranger.

The first year of life involves the essential psychosocial process of learning how to convert the innate herding tendency of any social species into a highly selective and discriminatory skill. It is this which is meant by communitive behaviour—interpersonal activity marked by a sense of unity, of being with another, but in which the relationship is willing and unforced, without loss of individuality. The child must not only be born, but he must be born into human society.

It would seem to be of particular biological significance that the infant has developed an elaborate sense of communion before he is able to walk. From 12 to 14 months or so onward, he is no longer dependent on the goodwill of his caregivers to provide him with interesting situations and objects, but can actively explore the environment for himself. An interesting developmental change which occurred some months previously is instrumental in ensuring the efficiency of this process. Up until six months of age or thereabouts the infant's world has been essentially centred on his mother, but from then on she is as it were moved sideways, and the infant explores his physical environment, the human world of artefact, of object and tool. His mother is an essential factor in this, and adults will always remain so. Once he can walk, and has learned to control a host of neuromotor problems involving body posture, balance, gait, and all this combined with effective use of the upper limbs in the development of different types of grasp, and the coordination between hand and eye in manipulative tasks, then he can expand enormously the efficiency and extent of his exploration. The potential for doing so, evidenced by grasping and reaching, and by avid visual scanning of his surroundings, has been present almost from the beginning. It is his locomotor abilities, first crawling then walking, running and climbing which enable him to exploit this desire to explore. Though exploration is such a notable feature of the developing child, it is held in tension with communion. The twelve-month-old likes to be constantly within sight and hearing of a familiar adult. Both now and later he is closely dependent upon the reassuring presence of such a person, and constantly returns to her. He is able to play contentedly alone, or if other children are in the vicinity, he will play near them, but is not yet able to play with them even at the age of two years. With his mother the picture is very different; he will follow her around the house, imitating her, searching for a duster or a broom so that he can be with her in her household activities; or he will drag a chair to the kitchen sink and help her (if that is the right word) do the washing-up and drying.

If the child, once he has acquired the necessary neuromotor coordination and skills to do so, is to explore, manipulate and inventory his world it is necessary for him to leave his mother. He will be obliged to separate himself from her not only bodily but also sensorily so that she is no longer available within his field of vision. This separation or detachment is opposed by his desire to return and be with her. The forces at work in this dynamic process will vary with age and with the state of the child; with the current state of the relationship between him and his mother; the sense of security and the intensity and permanence of the image, or internal representation he has attained of her; the familiarity of his surroundings; the novelty of the features within it; and the presence of intimidating features such as strangers or physical characteristics which are perceived as harmful. In consequence one sees in the young child a series of oscillations between leaving and returning, between exploratory and communitive behaviour.

2 The Emergence of the Objective World Sensory Processing and Motor Activity

The capability of speech to transmit thoughts of an almost infinite variety, and often with potent consequences, but in an intangible form with nothing connecting speaker and listener other than the air between them—or so it seems—gives it a magical quality. Language has become separated off and elevated above the perceptual and cognitive processes of mental activity so that in many people's minds it is autonomous, with its own rules and organization, owing nothing to the ordinary, mundane world. But this is to misunderstand the extraordinary power and versatility of cognitive activity, which is the source rather than the servant of language. If we want to examine the origins of language we must look—not at the child's first attempts to talk—but at the whole pattern of cognitive development in the child, from the moment he first opens his eyes on his new-born world.

The study of the young child as an activity in its own right is a curiously recent development. Mankind has a vast interest in itself but it is really only from the middle of this century that there has been a systematic attempt to explore the world of the infant. The picture has changed considerably and there is an extensive literature on child development, written from the very different, but complementary disciplines of psychology and medicine. Both these approaches are essential to our understanding of the child, and the two disciplines have much to learn from each other. In the account which follows the two strands intertwine, and are combined together and considered in so far as they are relevant to an understanding of the prelinguistic antecedents of language development. There is implicit in this the fundamental assumption that language can be looked at in this way, and does not arise *de novo* during the second year of life. In the interests of brevity it is not intended here to argue for or against this assumption. The absence of a formal defence will, it is hoped, subsequently be pardoned, as the relationships and dependencies between the structures of early language usage and features of cognitive processing become apparent. And if this in itself lacks sufficient conviction, the evidence provided by the different forms of language disorder should prove conclusive.

Amongst the wealth of material arising from the investigation of the child's early development, the writings of one particular person stand out as being preeminent, and it is to Jean Piaget that we will turn for an understanding of the early mental processes of the child. In his work "The Construction of Reality in the Child" published in 1934 (and in English in 1954), the processes by which the young child begins to make sense of his world are considered, in so far as anyone is able, from the point of view of the child. This is an astonishingly difficult concept to grasp, and a great deal of developmental work, both clinical and experimental, fails to distinguish between the viewpoint of the child and that of the person who is assessing or observing him. Even Piaget himself is frequently to be found commenting on what the child cannot do at any particular stage, though usually this is to trace and delineate the progress of some skill or behaviour he is examining. In the purely developmental approach it could be argued that there is no such thing as an ignorant or incapable child; these terms can only be applied by the less ignorant and more capable adult who is describing the child's activity or making various inferences about it. If one were to adhere strictly to the point of view of the child, one should look at him as if there is nothing he does not know, or cannot do, however little it is that he actually does know or manages to do.

Piaget's approach is an epistemological one, studying the growth of knowledge in the child, and in consequence totally relevant to our theme, in which it is asserted that knowledge of the objective world is an essential precursor of the development of language. It must be accepted that there are other theoretical viewpoints than that of Piaget, and for example one of the proponents of the stimulus-response school of cognitive development has reinterpreted aspects of Piaget's work in such terms (Berlyne, 1962). Bruner, who has contributed extensively on many aspects of child development, considers that intellectual growth can only be understood in the light of the psychological terms which mediate it and argues that the external pull of the child's environment plays a vitally important part in his mental growth. The nature of this growth is interpreted differently, being seen in the child's ability to represent the environment, and in his ability to integrate what has been experienced in the past, to the present and the future (Bruner, 1973). The child first learns to represent his world "enactively", that is through the motor responses which he acquires; this is later replaced or supplemented by "iconic" representation, relating to the child's ability to use images in place of the activity. The final form of representation is "symbolic", two basic features of which are category, and hierarchy, enabling the child to organize his world through symbols, and thus obtain a measure of freedom from its physical constraints. These and other theoretical positions are of considerable interest, and contribute to an understanding of the child's intellectual development, but it would be digressing too far from our purpose to examine them further. It is sufficient to note that certain aspects of Piaget's work, his approach to the stages and levels of development for instance, have not been universally accepted. Nevertheless, he provides a comprehensive view of the way in which the nature of the external world is grasped by the child, and it is supported by numerous observations which sum to a meticulous longitudinal description of early development.

Sensory and Perceptual Development

The child's growth of knowledge of the real world is divided by Piaget into a number of themes, the three most important for early development being object permanence, the spatial field, and causality, which together comprise the sensorimotor period of intellectual development, up until the second birthday. Each of these themes will be considered in turn (see Chapter 3), but an essential preliminary is to review the nature of the young child's sensory abilities, with particular reference to vision, hearing and touch, and the development of certain motor skills.

Vision

There is rapid development of visual function. The newborn child may lie quietly with his eyes open, and he shows clear evidence of seeing in that he will follow a moving hand, and especially the human face (Goren, Sarty, and Wu, 1975). He will turn his head towards a diffuse light, such as the window, and can fixate objects for an increasing period of time. Touwen (1976) found that by the end of the first month virtually all the infants in the series of 51 which he followed up through a wide range of developmental assessments were able to fixate a small, visually attractive object for at least a few seconds. One fifth of them could fixate the object for more than twenty seconds, and by 8 weeks this proportion had risen to two thirds. From about the third week onward the child is able to watch his mother's face during feeding or when she is talking to him with, as Sheridan (1975) says, an increasingly alert facial expression. The child is able to follow slowly moving objects from side to side, tracking them with his eyes. Touwen found that these visual pursuit movements, taking place through an arc of 30—60 degrees, could be demonstrated in at least eight percent of his children and some of them showed following movements in the neonatal period. By 20 weeks, over 80% showed pursuit movements through more than 90 degrees. The ability to fixate the object with both eyes so that true binocular vision is possible can be examined by watching the extent of convergence as an object is brought slowly nearer the child's face from a distance. At four weeks Touwen found that 75 per cent of the children showed no change of eye position for the approaching object, whilst from about 20 weeks, more than four fifths showed clear evidence of convergence which was maintained for more than a few seconds. This may be achieved by some children in the neonatal period, but its precise identification is difficult. Use is made of a technique which measures the reflection from the cornea of each eye, but there are unknown variables which affect the accuracy of the results (Slater and Findlay, 1972), and the technique may not be precise enough. So far we have been concerned with central vision, and the ability of the child to adjust the position of his eyes so that the image formed by the lens can fall on the foveal part of the retina. It is this part which is crucial for the discrimination of form, outline and detail. It is of the greatest importance that the child can detect movement and the occurrence of activity out of his direct line of sight, and the peripheral region of the retina has been specially adapted partly for this purpose. Though little is known of the way in which peripheral vision functions in the early stages of development it is highly sensitive to movement, to spatial location and the overall form of objects (Bronson, 1974).

Visual Perception

Children in the first weeks of life tend to scan their visual field along the horizontal axis. This means that a horizontal contour line much above or below the line along which he is traversing his visual field may well be missed, whereas vertically placed edges will be readily encountered. Haith (1976) does not consider this is due to any lack of sensitivity to horizontal contours because a horizontal edge lying along the line of the child's scan does engage scanning. His interpretation of the underlying mechanism of scanning is that the infant's visual behaviour is adjusted in such a way that there is maximal firing of the nerve cells in the visual cortex of the brain. The way in which children scan form shows an interesting change at about two months (Haith and Campos, 1977). Before this they scan the contour defining the overall form, or borders of high contrast, such as the chin-garment or hair-skin boundaries. From then on they scan internal features, which in the case of the face is mostly the eyes; and they are more sensitive to the organization of the detail of pattern in for instance the regularity of features, or the orientation of elements.

Visual Behaviour

It has already been noted that the child soon after birth is able to direct his gaze, and by one month eye movement is under increasingly smooth control. Not long after, he is beginning to show evidence of the perception of depth, with decrease of fixation time for objects which are much beyond 30 cm away (McKenzie and Day, 1972). By three months he is very alert visually , and showing particular interest in the human face, following the movements of his mother when she is nearby, and watching the movements of his hands and fingers (Sheridan, 1975). At six months he is intensely curious, looking at everything around him, and moving his head and eyes in every direction in order to study whatever catches his attention. He is able to follow closely the activities of those around him though they may be some distance away.

Hearing

The newborn and very young child responds to sound by blinking or opening his eyes to sudden sounds, and may move his eyes toward a sound. If the sound is loud, a generalized startle response is seen in which the arms stiffen and open out away from the body, with the hands open; the arms then slowly close back in over the chest, and he may screw his eyes up, grimace and start to cry. This pattern of response is not usually seen after three months though sudden loud sounds can be very distressing to the child long after. It is not the responses to loud noises which should be sought, but those to much quieter sounds such as the human voice when someone talks quietly to the child nearby, soothing him if he is beginning to fuss, or inducing smiling or quietening of activity as he listens, and he may vocalize or attempt to imitate certain voice sounds. It can be extremely difficult to interpret many of these responses because of the spontaneous activity and varying state of attention of the child. In clinical testing it is essential to determine the presence or absence of a hearing loss, and to quantify the threshold level in terms of frequency and intensity. Because of the ambiguity of many responses it is wise to rely only on the clear indication of hearing response given by the child's turning of his head and localization of the sound source. Touwen (1976) found that this did not occur in 80 per cent of the children in his series until six months, and not until nearly two months later for all the children without exception. As the test was not intended to measure the acuity of hearing the noise used was not quiet, but instead its stimulus level was well above threshold. Up until nearly three months there was only a diffuse reaction of the infant without clear evidence of orienting movements of the head, though some horizontal movements could be observed, and this clearly poses problems for any who attempt to measure aspects of hearing in the younger child.

Other indicators of hearing may be required if one is obliged to give an accurate and reliable estimate of auditory threshold in clinical medicine. Electrophysiological measures have become indispensable. The study of changes in the electroencephalographic recordings of brain activity evoked by auditory stimuli using long latency responses, of the order of 150 msec, have been used but their interpretation can give rise to considerable difficulty in this age group. At the other end of the latency time scale, the electrical activity induced in the auditory nerve (see Fig. 2.1. a) can be detected by an electrode passed through the tympanic membrane,with its tip lying in contact with the mucous membrane of the inner wall of the middle ear, near the round window. This procedure, known as transtympanic electrocochleography (E. Coch. G.) uses a train of rapidly recurring clicks as the sound stimulus in order to ensure maximal neural excitation (since a click has a wide frequency spectrum by virtue of its transient nature). Its use can only be justified for essential clinical purposes, because general anaesthesia is required in children. It is possible to follow the pattern of neural excitation up through the auditory pathways by means of a variation of this technique, in which the active electrode is placed further away from the cochlea on for instance the skin behind the ear. This procedure measures the brain-stem evoked response, and a complex of five or six waves is obtained, starting with the activity in the auditory nerve and ending with that in the inferior colliculus or medial geniculate body, see Fig. 2.1. b. Such techniques are now in widespread use for the clinical assessment of auditory threshold in difficult, often multiply handicapped children (Beagley, 1980, Gibson, 1978).

Certain naturally occurring activities have been made use of, where variation of the rate of activity can be shown statistically to be correlated with the reception of the sound. The heart rate has been found to be a useful indicator of this type (Eisenberg, 1976), the activity of the heart being monitored by an electrocardiograph machine. The complex wave pattern is reduced to a simple electrical signal which is then plotted in beats per minute, acceleration and slowing of the rate from the resting, interstimulus heart rate both serving as indicators of hearing under certain conditions. Another technique is to record electrically the mechanical de-

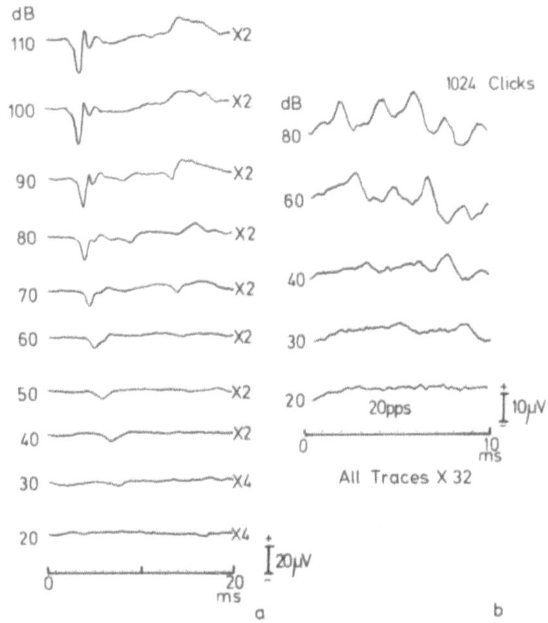

Fig. 2.1. Electrophysiological investigation of auditory function. *a* Transtympanic electrocochleography, *b* brainstem evoked response. Recordings of action potentials obtained in a one-year-old boy, showing normal auditory threshold. (By courtesy of H. A. Beagley, F.R.C.S. Nuffield Hearing and Speech Centre, Royal National Throat, Nose and Ear Hospital, London)

formations produced in the teat of a feeding bottle as the baby sucks on it, the sensing device being set up in such a way that only the more purposeful, vigorous sucks are recorded. Eimas (1974) established a baseline of high amplitude sucking and then presented an auditory stimulus in association with, or contingent upon each high amplitude suck. Typically, each child increased his sucking rate as the contingency was detected, but after a time this fell off as the novelty of the sound wore off. When it fell below a certain level the sound stimulus was changed and a new auditory pattern presented to the child, again contingent upon each more forceful suck. An increased rate of sucking associated with such a change of stimulus was taken to show that the child heard the sound as different from the one he had just previously been listening to, and that he could therefore discriminate between the two.

In order to overcome the ambiguity and observer error inherent in all procedures based on the visual detection of some overt response by the infant, equipment for semi-objective assessment of the relation of bodily activity to sound stimulus has been introduced, such as the Crib-o-gram designed by Simmons and Russ (1974). More recently Bennett (1979), taking advantage of the high information-processing capacity of the microprocessor, has designed a cradle in which the neonate's responses to sound can be evaluated in a precisely controlled manner, entirely instrumentally. The infant preferably aged 3–5 days old, is placed in the cradle: body movement, head turn and startle are detected through sensors incorporated in the mattress and the head rest, and respiratory activity through a transducer placed in a cotton band which is fitted round the upper abdomen over his clothing. No direct connections to the skin for any form of electrode placement are required. The apparatus constantly monitors patterns of bodily and respiratory activity. When a quiet 5 sec period is encountered, a 2600 Hz high pass broad band noise (effectively 2.6—4.5 kHz) at 80 dB can be produced or not, automatically, and the changes in motor activity and breathing contingent upon the sound stimulus are recorded. A series of checks are programmed into the operational routine so that random movements which might give false positive results are largely excluded. The apparatus is able to detect the various combinations of respiratory and general bodily activity more precisely than the trained observer and will probably prove sufficiently reliable to permit neonatal screening of hearing. Certain interesting features about its use have emerged. There is a clear, almost categorical difference in response between 70 dB and 80 dB SPL. The child, even at this age is extremely, and possibly selectively, responsive to the human voice, shown by the increase of activity. Because of the sensitivity of the apparatus it is possible to identify unduly restless and irritable or inert babies, and the cradle may prove of more general value, revealing abnormal patterns of neurological activity to the neonatal paediatrician.

Frequency of Sound Stimulus

The young child's sensitivity to pure tone stimuli has been a source of disagreement. Pure tones (which may be represented on oscilloscopes and graphic displays as sine waves and so referred to as sine wave or sinusoidal stimuli) have only the one frequency present in their sound spectrum, with no harmonics or other tones. Turkewitz, Birch, and Cooper (1972) considered that newborn children were insensitive to a wide range of loud (90 dB) pure tones but Kearsley (1973), using stimuli lasting more than one second, came to the opposite conclusion. A number of other electronically generated stimuli have been used, including white noise, in which all the frequencies of the sound spectrum are represented with uniform distribution of energy throughout the frequency range. This white noise may be given a tonal quality by filtering so that one may be left with a relatively narrow band of frequencies say 200 Hz wide, centred on a particular frequency. Apart from the pure tone, another periodic wave form that is frequently used is the square wave, but because of the sudden on- and off-changes of energy the sound produced has a complex harmonic structure,with many frequencies appearing in its spectrum. It has in consequence a more voice-like quality without resorting to the use of complex sound synthesizing equipment, but the experimental results have to be interpreted with extreme caution.

Leventhall and Lipsitt (1964) found that children could distinguish between square wave stimuli of 200 Hz and 1000 Hz lasting 10 sec, and Birns, Blank, Bridger, and Escalona (1965) showed that neonates could distinguish between 150 Hz and 500 Hz tones. Using long latency cortical evoked potentials, Lenard, von Bernuth, and Hutt (1969) found a larger amplitude response for 125 Hz than for 1000 Hz square wave stimuli. Eisenberg (1976) reports some interesting early observations on the differential effects of low and high frequency sounds. Dearborn (1910) noted that children as young as one week old found notes at the upper end of the piano's range to be disturbing, and Haller (1932) found a similar disturbing effect of high frequency pure tones to which there was little in the way of other overt response. Eisenberg concludes that there is unequivocal evidence for frequency discrimination during early life, and she considers that there is a qualitative difference between low and high frequency sounds as shown by the child's behaviour in response. Stimuli below 4000 Hz are two or three times more likely to induce a reaction, and low frequencies are more effective in inhibiting a child's distress. High frequencies on the other hand will cause rather than reduce distress, and will induce a freezing response; this can be sufficiently powerful a reaction to inhibit a Moro reflex momentarily.

Duration of Sound

Keen (1964) found that sound stimuli lasting for 10 sec were more effective than those lasting 2 sec in changing the pattern of sucking in the newborn. Using square wave stimuli varying in duration from 2 sec to 30 sec, and assessing the response of newborn children by the increase of heart rate, Clifton, Graham, and Hatton (1968) found there was progressive increase in rate up to 10 sec, after which it began to fall off. Eisenberg (1965) found that there was a more or less direct relationship between the duration of pure tones and filtered bands of noise, and the extent of the child's responses between 300 msec and 5 sec. The ability to process accurately the duration of sounds and intervening pauses, and the temporal patterns produced thereby are of fundamental importance as a preliminary to the perception of the rhythm and syllabic structure of speech.

Hearing Behaviour

There is a widespread tendency to picture the primary hearing skill of the child as the ability to detect very quiet sounds. This overvalues the role of sensation at the expense of perception. Those who work with the hearing impaired have at their disposal a fundamentally important measuring device in the form of the pure tone audiometer. It is an instrument for generating sounds of a highly specialized nature, in which the energy is located virtually at a single frequency, as happens with a well constructed tuning fork. In order to assess hearing, pure tones are selected, usually an octave apart, in the range of frequencies from 125 Hz–8000 Hz; at each frequency the intensity of the sound is decreased in 10 dB or 5 dB steps until the listener can no longer hear that tone. The investigation should be carried out in a properly sound-treated room and measures the threshold of hearing. This sensation level reflects the threshold of excitation in appropriate groups of hair cells arranged along the basilar membrane of the inner ear, and their related sensory nerve fibres. The threshold of sensation obtained in this way provides a highly meaningful statement about certain aspects of auditory function. We need however, to know much more about the processing of sound in the auditory pathways, including such features as the discrimination of fine differences of pitch and loudness, the nature of discrimination of more intricately structured sounds, or the detection of specific patterns at various levels of organizational complexity.

The pure tone audiogram's ubiquity as a test procedure in clinical practice has resulted in the conceptualization of hearing as the ability to detect a very quiet sound against a background of silence. Though of great value this is a totally artificial concept. Complete silence and pure tones are not natural features of human auditory space. There is never a time that the human embryo has not been exposed to noise. From the time before the development of the sensory apparatus of the ear, the embryo has been immersed in all the internal noise of his mother's abdominal cavity. Once the child is born the range of sounds increases immeasurably. His problem is not one of detecting a sound against a background of silence. It never has been. His problem is to isolate or to detect amongst the array of sounds reaching him from all directions, that particular group or sequence of sounds which has meaning for him. How he does this, how he begins to organize sounds and categorize them as "same" or "different", how he begins to recognize them, classify and attach significance to them—about all this we are woefully ignorant. Some information is becoming available for the crucially important sounds of speech.

The Perception of Speech and Speechlike Sounds

Acoustically, speech consists of an extremely complex series of patterns of sound, in which there may be several component parts present at any one time and in one or more of which relatively brief but perceptually significant changes occur. Moffitt (1971) investigated the ability of children aged 5–6 months to perceive the difference between a complex sound in which a falling or a rising tone preceded a steady state lasting 250 msec. He synthesized two consonant-vowel syllables in which the only difference was this transition of frequency in the resonant band of frequencies known as the second formant. The steady state was held at 1075 Hz and was preceded by a tone which either started at 2078 Hz and fell, or at 846 Hz and rose to 1075 Hz in a time of 55 msec. The first sound is heard as "ga" and the second as "ba". The sounds were given in a series of groups and the effect on the heart rate was used as the indicator of response. The end result was that if a long run of "ba"-like sounds was followed by "ga" there was little effect, but if the order was reversed there was a significant slowing of heart rate as the stimulus changed from "ga" to "ba". Morse (1972) used the sucking patterns in children aged 40–54 days to investigate the same perceptual feature, and also the child's ability to detect the difference of the fundamental frequency contour of the syllable. He concluded that the children did detect these differences. Eimas and his co-workers (1971) had used this technique earlier to investigate the child's ability to detect the onset of voicing in plosive consonant-vowel combinations. In his experiments he changed the voice onset time by 20 msec, and concluded that his groups of one-month and four-month-olds could perceive the difference between "b" and "p". "The evidence thus indicates that the mechanisms responsible for detecting differences in voicing are sensitive not to absolute differences in voicing, but rather to whether the particular values of voicing being discriminated represent the same or different phonetic feature values" (Eimas, 1974). By this is meant that the child responds to the difference in voice onset time in a way that shows he is discriminating not between progressive degress of difference but across a category boundary, when a physical change in quantity results in a perceptual change of quality.The sound is no longer heard as "b" but as "p", the two being placed as it were in different categories on the basis of some discriminable contrast.

Whilst accepting the experimental results, it is difficult to accept the conclusions that these very young children are born with the ability to make phonetic distinctions, meaning that they are processing the sounds in a linguistically relevant manner from birth. A more parsimonious explanation is that the neural structures which comprise the auditory pathways include a series of pattern detection features, one of which might well be for instance the property to respond selectively to a brief tone of falling frequency, its upper and lower limits being preset. There is nothing in this which runs counter to the findings of neurophysiologists working for example on pattern detectors in vision. Similarly Fourcin (1978) considers that the discriminations are sensory rather than phonetic and goes on:

"It does not follow, however, that the ability to categorize speech sounds contrastively, so that communication ability is achieved in a particular language environment, can be innate. This is a higher skill which must be learnt from experience, and which could well in part depend on an innate auditory ability to process prominent acoustic pattern traits."

The time course of language development entirely supports this conclusion. The child's ability to detect linguistically meaningful patterns of sound which are based on the segmental features of consonants and vowels does not emerge until nine months of age or so, when he first begins to recognize and respond appropriately to certain simple word patterns such as "bye bye". There are features of the spoken voice which the child has been responding to long before this. Fourcin (1978) gives the example of a four week-old who produces a sequence of a falling tone, a level tone and then a slightly rising tone which is reinforced by the mother who imitates it in a subtly modified way, which is then immediately repeated by the infant.

The necessity for a long apprenticeship in speech perception, even allowing for the fact that the infant nervous system has built into it from before birth a sensory processing ability which permits the detection of certain acoustic features, suggests the probability of a developmental progression. Fourcin (1979) has outlined the likely stages as being—first the ability to detect the presence or absence of voice; then the ability to perceive changes in pitch of the voice; this is followed by perception of changes in the second and third formants and the relationship between the changes in these two formants; and finally there is the elaboration of the auditory schemata based on the child's perception of acoustic pattern cues which enable him to contrast and so to categorize all the segmental features of a spoken utterance. If we take as a guide the ages at which first 50 per cent and then 90 per cent of children use for themselves certain consonants as in Fig. 2.2. we may, in general rather than specific terms, assume that this developmental sequence follows and reflects the sequence of their perception in the mediation of language. A clear distinction must be made between linguistic and pre-linguistic patterns of vocal activity (see Chapter 4).

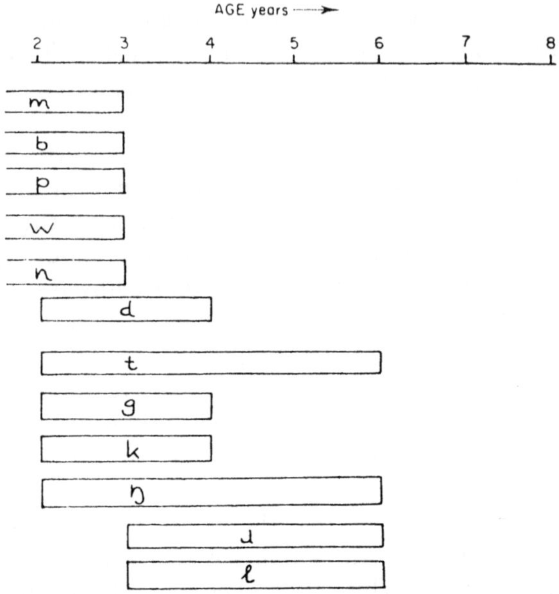

Fig. 2.2. Consonant acquisition. This summary of English consonant developmental studies is based on a convenient representation introduced by Sander (1972). The left-hand bar for each closed box corresponds to the age at which 50% of the children studied use the sound (ideally this should be a contrastive use); the right-hand bar corresponds to the 90% age. Initial, medial and final position occurrences have been averaged. /h/ has been omitted; grouping follows phonetic class. From Fourcin, A. J. (1978): Acoustic Patterns and Speech Acquisition. In: The Development of Communication (Waterson, N., Snow, C., eds.)

Motor Development

Control of the Position and Movement of the Head

The young child, if he is to develop the use of his visual and auditory abilities, must acquire control of the position and movements of his head. It is the platform on which the eyes and ears are mounted and they are integral features of it. The head is connected by the neck flexibly to the trunk of the body and the lower limbs, and these combine to provide a continuously adjusted, stable but mobile structural support. This requires a whole series of incessantly active, meticulously inter-coordinated control mechanisms ensuring precise regulation of directional and tracking systems so that the distance sensors of hearing, and especially of sight, can be brought to bear on the object of attention. As adults we have long since been accustomed to directing our eyes to what is happening in the world around and at our fingertips, and it is difficult to think it could be otherwise, until the necessity to acquire a particular skill reminds us that even now our abilities are not necessarily fully developed in this direction. The trainee ear, nose and throat surgeon, obliged to use a lamp or light-reflecting mirror attached to his forehead in order to ensure adequate illumination, has the greatest difficult in coordinating the movements of his eyes and hands with that of his head, so that he can unerringly direct the beam of light to the tips of his instruments. Until the child can move his head in exactly the direction he requires, at the appropriate rate and in a smoothly coordinated fashion without tremor or jerkiness, the eyes and ears cannot be used as effective probes, sampling the environment and conveying sensory data to the brain for further analysis. This control develops rapidly and by six months or shortly after the child, held sitting, is able to hold his head firmly erect, and to turn it so that he can look from side to side. In order to do so he has had to integrate neural activity originating in the semicircular canals and otolith organs of the vestibular apparatus with that arising in the proprioceptive pathways relating to muscle tension and stretch in the various groups of muscles surrounding the head and neck and running between them, and in the nerve endings situated in the capsules of the joints of the cervical spine and at the base of the skull.

Probably the first evidence which can be elicited of vestibular otolith activity is in the use of the head-drop method to demonstrate the Moro reflex in the newborn. With the infant lying on his back, the examiner's hand supports his head and drops it minimally; as the child's head drops back the reflex response occurs. With increasing control of the head and neck musculature during the first three months of life the reflex disappears. Similarly the head lag which occurs so prominently when the newborn is pulled to sit up from a lying position has virtually disappeared by three months. If the child is placed prone on his front, he is able to lift his head and to keep it lifted for some few seconds from one month onward. The situation is very different when the child is placed supine, on his back. Touwen (1976) found that none of the children in his series were able to lift their heads during the first three months, and that 80 percent were not able to lift up their heads for at least five seconds until eight months had elapsed. Clearly the strength of the muscle groups responsible for extension of the head and cervical spine is much greater than the flexor musculature. Touwen considers that the ability to lift the head whilst supine reflects in addition the differentiation of vestibular mechanisms which enable the child to orient his head in space. The importance of the position of the head in relation to the rest of the body can also be seen in the movements by which the child rolls over; this movement starts with rotation of the head and the body follows. Some children are able to roll from lying on their backs over onto their fronts or vice versa by three months though the majority have not succeeded in doing this until six months.

If the child is to be in a position to explore his surroundings, he must be able to sit. The parents are able to anticipate this stage by sitting the child up with the secure support of cushions so that he can look around and take an interest in what is happening, rather than staring at the ceiling during his waking hours. In the development of sitting, from being unable to without support (Touwen, 1976), the major change occurs at eight months, and from shortly thereafter 80 percent could at the least sit free for some seconds, whilst at 11 months this proportion could sit unaided for over a minute. If the sitting position is to be an effective base from which to explore his surroundings it must be stable, with the child able to control his balance whilst carrying out various search and reach activities. Good balance was found in over 80 percent of Touwen's series by the age of one year, with the ability to watch an object move through an arc which extended to 90 degrees each side of the midline.

Touch, Reach and Grasp

There is unfortunately all too little known about the developmental progress of tactile sensation, though precise control of the hands and fingers is of vital importance to virtually all human activity. Speech itself is highly dependent upon the ability to monitor the location and extent of contact points between say, the tip of the tongue and alveolar ridge, and the degree of pressure exerted and released during the formation of various of the consonants must also be controlled in part by tactile sensors in the epithelium of the lips, tongue and palate.

The sense organs in the skin of the finger tips which permit recognition of objects by feel and manipulation are to be found in two main sites. Weissner's receptors are found tightly coupled to the deep under-surface of the epidermis and are also found in the lips and the tip of the tongue, important for the young child who is constantly referring everything to his mouth. They develop just about the time of birth (Williams and Warwick, 1975, p. 798). The Paccinian corpuscle is found in the deeper, more loosely arranged layer of the skin, and is sensitive to rapidly rising deformation in which high frequency vibration occurs, of the order of 100—300 Hz. The ridged fingerprint structure of the skin coupled with the rate of movement of the finger tips across the surface being touched and felt will be important features of the stimulus complex. Another, important type of sensory receptor is the Ruffini ending, found in joint capsules, and relevant here because of the information conveyed on the positions of the fingers and their spatial relationship, one to the other. Through the patterns of activation of these various sensory endings a complex neural pattern of activity is set up which is collated and enters consciousness to convey awareness of what it is we are feeling, its surface texture, consistency and shape.

The Use of the Hands

The overall outline of the development of the use of the hands is derived from the series of age related descriptions given by Sheridan (1975) and Drillien (1977, p. 56 et seq). In the first month of life large, jerky movements of the upper limbs occur; at rest the hands are held closed with the thumbs turned in across the palms. A reflex grasping movement can be demonstrated at this stage by pushing in a finger or pencil from the side of the hand under the fingers. The resulting grip is strong enough that one may lift the child's body through it. The reflex disappears by about three months, and in doing so the way is prepared for the purposive use of the hands. At this age the child plays with his hands and fingers, bringing them together in front of him and watching their movements. He may hold an object, such as a rattle, for a short while but at eight weeks is not able to look at it at the same time. A month later he is able to do so briefly, limb movements are smoother and the hands are held more loosely open. By six months he has gained good control of limb movement so that he can reach out for objects, often with both hands, which he usually succeeds in grasping and then manipulates by shaking or passing from hand to hand, looking as he does so, and takes everything to his mouth for further examination. In considering purposeful, goal-directed use of the arms and hands, Touwen (1976) found that hand regard and finger play was achieved by the majority at three months; a month later they could attempt to grasp an object, though not necessarily successfully until six months or so when they could reach for and hold an object with one hand. The next stage, in which an object is held in the second hand, without dropping the object in the first, shows a wide age scatter but the majority have achieved this by about eight months. He concludes that this type of activity is essentially mediated by non-cortical brain structures, more specifically the basal ganglia, the brain stem and the cerebellum. The development of a steady sitting posture which appears at the same time is most probably mediated through the same neurological structures. Fully differentiated manual ability, in which the motor cortex is involved in its organization, is described as occurring when the child is able to accept a third object whilst holding an object in each hand. This is usually accomplished by the child transferring one of the objects already held to the other hand, thus freeing a hand to take the newly offered one. A number of children were able to achieve this complex task before nine months, though the 80 percent figure was not reached until 14 months.

From nine months on the child shows a great interest in handling objects, turning them over and examining them attentively. He pokes at small objects with his index finger and is beginning to point at more distant objects. Control of grasp is such that it is difficult as yet to put held objects down, and the child resorts to dropping them or releasing them by pressing down against a firm surface. The development of grasp has naturally attracted a good deal of interest, and it passes through a number of well-defined stages. In the first stage the child uses the whole of the palmar surface of the hands and fingers (not to be confused with the reflex grasp which will have disappeared by this age). The details of developmental progress are shown in Fig. 2.3. The full maturation of grasp is dependent upon the close integration of highly differentiated fine finger movements with the sensory activity which accompanies and monitors them, and this requires the mediation of the sensorimotor areas of the cortex. Touwen speculates that pointing might mark the transition between non-cortical and cortically mediated grasping mechanisms.

With the appearance of the mature form of pincer grasp the way is open for the child to acquire and perfect a wide range of manipulative skills. Skill as defined by Elliott and Connolly (1974) includes an ability to achieve defined goals. It is to some extent synonymous with efficiency, so that a sequence of actions is organized into a purposeful plan which is executed with economy. The overall organization involves the use of sub-routines, basic units of well-practised activity, which are combined together into more complex patterns in a specific sequence. So there develops the notion of a schema or programme, a rule-based syntax as it were, of sequentially ordered acts. By this means a relatively restricted number of subroutines may be combined together in differing concurrent and sequential patterns to achieve a vast variety of skilled operations.

With the advent of standing, and more particularly walking, the child's spatial world acquires another dimension, in which his urge to explore and his curiosity can eventually gain full expression. His rapidly increasing physical abilities do not however afford him limitless freedom, because there are marked psychological

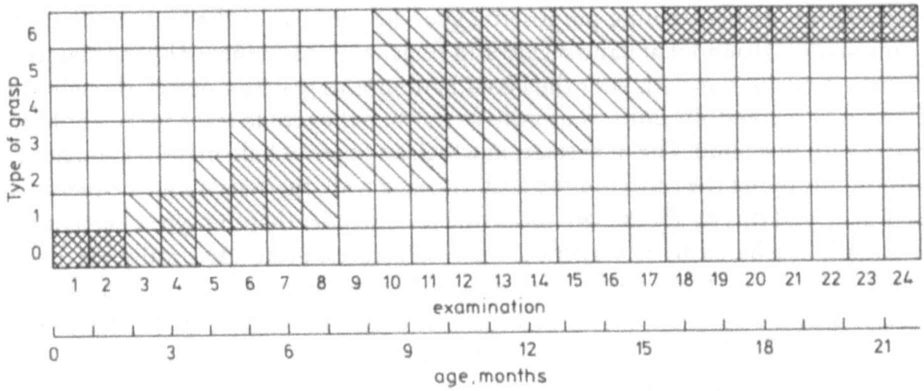

Fig. 2.3. Type of voluntary grasping. After Touwen, B. (1976): Neurological Development in Infancy

0 No grasping of the object
1 Palmar grasp: when grasping the infant used the whole palmar surface of hands and fingers
2 Radial palmar grasp: the infant mainly used the radial half of his palm, including thumb and index finger
3 Scissor grasp: the infant grasped the object between the volar surfaces of his extended thumb and index finger
4 Inferior pincer grasp: the infant grasped the object between the tip of his index finger and the volar side of his thumb
5 Pointing: the infant appeared unable to grasp, but he pointed and eventually touched the object with an extended index finger ("tipping"). Sometimes this pointing was followed by an inferior or good pincer grasp
6 Pincer grasp: the infant grasped the object neatly between the tips of index finger and thumb

Level of ability achieved by 100 per cent of children at that examination

Level(s) of ability achieved by at least 80 per cent of children

Upper and lower limits of ability achieved by remaining 20 per cent

constraints, such as attachment to parents and anxiety in the presence of strangers or in strange places. The transition from the age when 80 percent of the children could not stand till the same proportion were able to achieve a standing position whilst holding on took place between 9 and 13 months (Touwen, 1976). His findings for the ability to walk unaided for a few paces show that 10 percent could manage this at 13.5 months, whilst the 90 percent figure was not reached until 18 months. This seems somewhat slow; Sheridan and Drillien agree that the 15 month-old is usually able to walk alone with uneven steps, the arms held up for balance; whilst at 18 months he is walking well and able to stop and start safely. The Bayley scale of infant development gives the median age as 11.8 months (Bayley, 1969), so there is considerable variation in the recorded estimates of this activity. At 18 months the child is exploring his environment energetically and with understanding, pushes and pulls large toys and other objects around the floor , often carries favorite toys around with him and shows increasing manipulative skill with spoon and cup, can pick up and carefully release bricks to put two or three on top of one another and has ceased taking everything to his mouth.

The Emergence of the Objective World The World Made Sensible 3

Up to now we have been considering the child from the point of view of the observer. This may be one who intrudes as little as possible in the activities and interactions of the child with the people and objects in his normal surroundings, or the psychologist or paediatrician who deliberately intervenes to carry out some carefully controlled manipulation of the child or his environment. It is necessary to go a stage further and make an attempt to understand the world of the child as it is perceived by him. That it is possible to do so may be made clear by an example. A child who is handed what is in fact a small, shaped piece of wood and plastic will demonstrate that he has recognized the object for what it is meant to be by the way he handles it, as in Fig. 3.1 he tries to turn the tap on the kitchen sink, and subsequently explores the cupboards underneath. If he had not recognized the object as a representation or symbol his actions would be incomprehensible, and indeed he would not have been able to carry them out. This is not because of any physical limitation, but because he had not yet reached the appropriate level of cognitive development which enabled him to perceive the small object in his hand as a representation of the sink unit in his mother's kitchen. It is on the basis of this sort of inference that Piaget has been able to reconstruct the child's world. The pages which follow provide a summary of the three fundamental concepts of the object, space and causality which Piaget (1954) considers essential to a naive, but developing understanding of the external world. It is only after these concepts develop in the mind of the child that he can begin to understand and to use spoken language.

The Object

The nature of the object is given pride of place in the child's material world, and neither space nor causality can be understood until this concept is grasped. It may be added that this is a two way process; the object cannot be fully comprehended

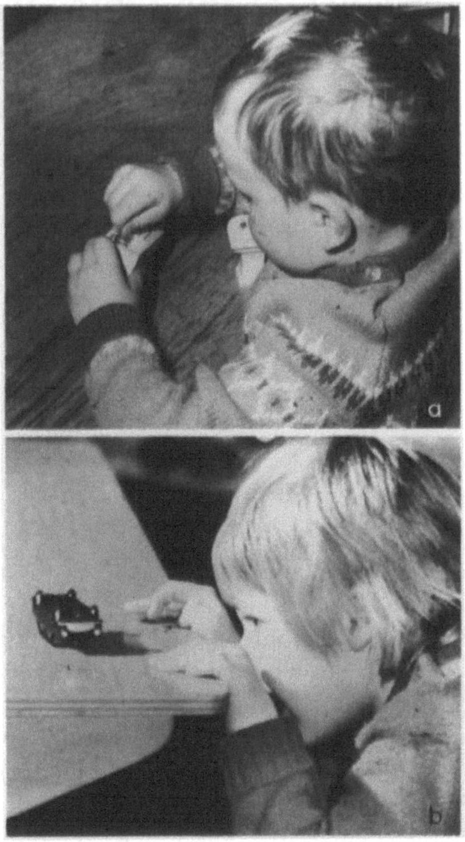

Fig. 3.1. *a* A child aged 20 months showing by his attempt to turn the tap on the miniature sink unit that he has recognized and understood the representational nature of the object he is holding, *b* A retarded and autistic child aged 3½ years unable to recognize the object in front of her as a miniature car

until the space which contains it, and the effects which various forces and actions have on it, are also understood. The three concepts develop together through progressively more advanced stages, intertwined and dependent on each other.

In the early months, the object cannot be separated from the action which obtains it, whether this be the hand which grasps or the gaze which holds it. Though the young child might appear to the observer to be engaged in searching, it is rather that the child has the expectation that his activity will result in recreating the tactile or visual image. This emphasis on the priority of action receives support from Hamburger (1976). In his review of the developmental history of the motor neurone he emphasizes the primacy of spontaneous activity, which must not be confused with reactivity or response. So he develops the notion of the creativity of movement, and quotes Goethe's Faust "In the beginning was the Act...", a precise transliteration of Saint John's "In the beginning was the Word...".

If one accepts Piaget's thesis it might be thought that object recognition would not be possible until some much later time than the child actually demonstrates his ability at this. Sensory schemas are however already developing which enable a comparison to be made between them and the images brought forth by the child's activity, recognition being the conformity of the internal schema to the sensory image presented to him by his eyes or his hands as he perceives the object.

By three months he is beginning to grasp what he sees, and to look at what he touches. There is an early integration of input from different sensory pathways, and this contributes to solidifying the child's object world. As control of visual tracking improves it is possible to follow quickly moving objects and this further adds to their permanence. Some object which has been dropped is too difficult to follow and so it disappears out of his world; after the age of five or six months the child will search for it, first if he has dropped it himself and then if some other person has dropped it. Similarly in the following of objects moving horizontally across his line of vision rather than vertically, a greater sense of permanence is implied in the way that from six months or so, the child will follow the line of an object's trajectory when the object itself can no longer be seen. Tactile permanence precedes visual, and the child will systematically follow with his hand and try to find some toy which he has only felt and not seen. At seven or eight months the child is beginning to be able to reconstruct the whole object when only part of it can be seen, and he will seek actively to regain it so long as it remains partly visible. If the object is completely hidden it has vanished and no search is made, even if the object is covered up in some way only just before the child actually grasps it. Furthermore Gratch and Landers (1971) found that if the cover was dropped a little late, just as the object had been grasped, the six month-old would not retrieve it, and this continued until a median age of 7 months 18 days (7.6 months). From about six or seven months the child has been able to remove say a pillow from off his own face so that he can look and see, but does not remove the cover over some object if the object is made completely invisible by it. During this stage of development objects persist longer because the child is able to control his own actions more skilfully, but the action and the object remain closely inter-related. The emotional content of the activity becomes apparent through the child's desire to continue the action and make the object persist, and by the tension which accompanies his efforts or in his disappointment when it disappears.

Active search starts at about 9 months so that the child will remove an adult's hand deliberately covering and hiding something, but difficulties remain. Though it is now possible to find something where it was seen to be hidden (label this—site A) the child cannot find the object at site B even though he was watching carefully all the time the object was transferred from A to B. As soon as it is hidden from view at B the child returns to A and searches for it there. Exactly the same behaviour can be seen when a sound producing object is made to produce its sound in a new place—the child looks to where it usually makes its sound. This is known as the $A\overline{B}$ (A, not B) error. Gratch (1976) found the median age for this to be 8.1 months, the search directly at B not appearing until 9 months 8 days (9.3 months). What the error shows is that the object itself is not yet completely separated off from the child's action in searching, and from its usual or initial location in space. It isn't that there are multiple objects but that the object and the place it occupies are bound together, i.e. "teddy-on-bed" or "ball-under-armchair", the image of the object evoking for the child more than the object alone.

Once the child can accurately follow a series of visible displacements of an object and still find it in the right place as it is moved from one hiding place to another, the way is made clear for the next and final stage of development of object concept. By this time the child has built up an image of the object as having a considerable degree of permanence, and has learned to separate the object from his own actions, so that it exists "objectively" as it were, in its own right and independent of him. The process is continued and completed when the child is able to follow a series of removals or displacements of an object which have been concealed in some way. This might be achieved by putting a toy in the hand, putting the hand under a cushion without letting the child see the object and removing it again, or transferring the toy from one hand to the other behind one's back. Concealment can also be achieved by putting an object in a box, having first wrapped it up, and then hiding the box. Piaget's children could successfully track the various invisible displacements of an object in this way by the age of 15—18 months. There are two important implications. The object has now been freed completely from perception and action alike; it exists in its own three dimensional right and without the child having any chance to see or touch it. Associated with this complete objectivity the child is able to retain an effective, long term representation, a multi-sensory image or model, of the object in his mind which does not depend on any sensory reminder. The ability to represent people and things which can no longer be directly experienced through any of the senses is an essential step towards understanding the world and making sense of it.

Space

It is important for the child to understand the spatial relationships which exist between various objects, between these and the various salient features and fixed landmarks of his surroundings, and between all these and his own body, when he is still and as he moves about. Space is derived from what it contains and what takes place in it. Movements, and especially the child's own movements, are particularly important in the construction of space. From the beginning the child's activity creates space, though this space is not one but many. It may be buccal (or oral) space, with the child's reflex search for the breast; this is elaborated in the second month as coordination of activity between hand and mouth begins to appear; and at three months as the child takes things to his mouth. This is not connected with visual space, and the child does not look at what he is grasping and putting in his mouth. Visual space is developing, as we have seen in the child's ability to follow various movements of objects. Auditory and tactile space are shown by the rather vague early search of the eyes and sideways movements of the head on hearing a sound, or the patting, searching movements of the hands when a grasped object has been lost.

As the child brings objects to his mouth, he learns how to control their orientation in space. At first this is largely fortuitous but by five months the increasing coordination between hand and mouth, or one might say the increasingly close connection between tactile (or manual) and buccal space, ensures more effective placing so that the child can find the most pleasing aspect of the object to put in his mouth and suck. With further coordination involving the use of vision, the child will more purposefully turn the object round, a rattle for instance, so that he can mouthe and suck the handle which he has seen. Now that he is able to look at what he is doing, the child sees the contact of his hands with the object and in a real sense begins to see himself act. The result is much greater coordination of the various forms of space, but space remains essentially defined and delimited by his own activity, as the medium in which he is able to carry out his actions. At 6—7 months there is near space, in which he is able to reach for and grasp an object, though he is not always successful in this and may well reach out for objects which are beyond his manual space; and there is distant space, in which objects are remote and inaccessible. He can only locate objects in relation to himself and as a function of his own movements so that space remains centred on him and on his activities.

The child's understanding of space increases as he furnishes it with objects which are more permanent. Solid objects acquire a constant size and shape despite the many differing visual appearances due to their distance from the eyes or their orientation in space. The child in the last quarter of the first year will spend some considerable time simply looking at an object in his hand, moving it nearer and further away. The tactile sensation remains constant despite the change of distance or of the position of the object in space as he moves or rotates it. This meticulous appraisal suggests that it is almost as if objects, some of which are very familiar to him, are being seen for the first time. The same applies to the fixed features of his environment; the child thoughtfully examines his surroundings as he moves himself around by altering his posture and the position of his head, by for example leaning from one side to the other. As he does so, he acquires a greater sense of depth, and its arrangement in receding planes, and becomes aware of "in front of" and "behind" through the effect of parallax, in which nearer objects move more than objects further away as the head moves at a right angle to the line of vision. Some objects, and especially people, are understood as moving in their own right, quite independent of any action of his, and he is now able to grasp the spatial basis for these movements. A child follows an adult with his head and eyes as he passes behind his pram, then quickly turns to look behind him on the other side as the person comes back into view.

In the months after his first birthday, with further improvement of coordination between hand and eye, the child is able to explore the relationships which exist between different objects as they occupy zones of space which are nearer to him or further away. He will put things down on the floor and study the various arrangements which they make and then move them, showing that he is interested in them for their own sake rather than specifically in relation to himself, as has been the case in the past up till now. Things are put on top of one another, like bricks, or a tray on a bowl; things are incessantly put into one another, such as pebbles and small objects placed in containers and taken out again one by one: the container is not emptied all in one go until two or three months later. The child is aware of his own movements in relation to objects occupying space, such as items of furniture which he has to walk round, or as he goes round mother's back to get something she has hidden behind her.

The ability to understand the relationships of objects to one another develops from about 18 months. Space is now a motionless environment in which the child is located and in which his actions take place—and in which the actions of others take place independently of himself. He has come to see himself as an object whose spatial relationships must be looked at in the same way as other objects, rather than himself occupying a uniquely privileged position in space in relation to everything else. The efforts of a child to retrieve a ball which he has thrown under a settee and which he can no longer see, let alone reach, show that he can retain in his mind the movements of the ball and the position it now probably occupies in space. The movements which he must make to regain possession of it are very different. He might have to move past various obstructions such as other items of furniture, which may take him further away from the ball, until he can get behind the settee where the ball has come to rest. He has represented to himself the invisible movements of the ball in order to achieve this. The internal process of the representation of movement, in which the invisible is made clear to the mind's eye, is an essential step because it is frequently not possible to see all the various movements which take place, nor is it possible to understand the apparent movements of objects in relation to one another as the child moves his head or his body. Furthermore, in order fully to understand these movements, objects must exist in a spatial dimension which is independent of him, and in which he himself moves as another object.

The grasp of relationships, in this case spatial, is important for all cognitive activity. The true nature of space does not reside simply in the sensory information the child obtains from his eyes, his hands or his hearing but from the intellectual activity which processes this information and builds up a working model of the real world. This ability is well developed by the second birthday, and remains a prime feature of human cognitive activity throughout life. We never cease trying to make more sense out of the world we live in and our place in it, whether physically or metaphysically.

Cause and Effect

For the child in the first month or two of his life the world is a collection of events arising out of his own activities and there is no causality apart from him. The things which he sees and touches and hears result from his activity and the stimuli or images received sustain and extend it in their turn, such as the milk at feed time which is the results of his action of sucking. At this stage every phenomenon may be considered in this way, and cause and effect are condensed into one. It will be recalled that there is no common space, but rather that each activity occupies its own space. With the limited information processing capacity of the infant, activities can only be attended to in one space at a time, so that the child who is engaged visually is apparently deaf until his visual attention is modified, either spontaneously or by the action of his mother. This limitation of perceptual processing is not peculiar to the child but is a relative matter and characteristic of human activity at all ages (Broadbent, 1958).

The appearance of an interest in causal relations begins with the child's increasing awareness that certain of his movements result in certain effects. When for instance he moves in his pram and a rattle attached to some part of it makes a noise, or if he is holding a rattle and moves his hand, it is not the object which causes the sound but his activity.

The child's discovery of an association between what he has just done and the visual or auditory effect may result in a smile. Because of this Watson (1973) describes the detection of contingency as being pleasurable to the child, the source of pleasure being his discovery of a connection between some event and his own activity. In view of the intense curiosity which the human shows about his world it is interesting that evidence for its emotional basis is manifested so young, in circumstances which rule out the possibility of the child's mother as the cause of the smile. This smile is not social but cognitive in origin. The hands become increasingly effective tools, obeying his desires to grasp and hold, and this starts when at three months or so he looks at his hands and plays with them. As coordination between hand and eye develops and he sees the contact of his hands on objects and the results which he can produce, so the underlying motivation of desire and sense of effort become distinct from the specific effects of his activity. By eight months or so he studies very carefully the movements of his hands and other parts of the body which are beginning to be seen as having function and purpose.

As for people, they too are seen at first as an extension of his activity; it is his action, his cry, which is effective in bringing his mother to his side if he is hungry or uncomfortable. Even later this sequence of events is not the relation of effect to cause. When at 8–9 months he expects to see his mother on hearing the door open, there is no reason to consider that he thinks the movement of the door is caused by his mother. But important differences are emerging between the way he treats causality in the physical world and in the world of people. People are clearly much more active, and personal contact plays an essential role in the progressive construction of his world. They are the first objects to exist in their own right and they show their own spontaneous activity. The child shows he has reached the stage of recognizing this by the way he expectantly watches his mother, waiting for her to act without any further initiative on his part. Causality becomes detached from the child's actions alone, and is identified as being located independently in people, and especially in his mother. Nevertheless, people remain for some considerable time longer subservient to his desires and activities, and it is difficult to see how it could be otherwise since this is a biological function and necessity of parenthood.

The first clear evidence of the child's grasp of causal effort and the effect it produces is shown in his manual activity as he pulls objects towards himself or pushes them along; the importance of the contact of the hand with the object is learned during this type of activity. The required result is not obtained merely by waving a hand, or arching and moving the body agitatedly when the child wants something to happen; these were actions he resorted to at an earlier stage as if they could in some magical way produce the desired effect. There is a tendency to revert to this more primitive notion of causality whenever the desire or necessity for the required result exceeds the child's ability to effect it. And it is not only in children that irrational behaviour of this type is resorted to in the effort to achieve ends which are beyond the individual's or the local community's reach and power. The child at 8 months can show his understanding of the efficacy of others by for instance putting his mother's hand to an object in order to make it swing, and leaving it there in the expectation that she will then carry on the desired action. Or he may put his finger to her lips in order to make her produce the same sound again after she has stopped singing. He is no longer the sole source of causality, but is instead, as it were, sharing it with others. His action now merely releases the effectiveness of his mother's hand or lips which are the true causal agents.

Soon after this stage is seen, the child treats physical objects with the same gentleness, beginning to realize they are acted on by forces outside himself, which he can only release. By 11—12 months he will very carefully push an object along to the edge of a table so that it will fall of its own accord, and does not have to be thrown down. People are seen as much more autonomous; they no longer have to be acted upon through some activity of the child, but it is now sufficient to wait and they will carry out the desired action. The child who wants a box opened will simply put it in his mother's hand, and wait. The spatial dimension of causality is discovered by the child learning the use of intermediary objects which will act between his hands and the desired object itself. He pulls the cushion, or whatever the supporting object is, in order to obtain the toy or biscuit placed on it which would otherwise be beyond his grasp. A stick can no longer be banged about erratically if he wants to knock something over, but instead precise physical contact has to be achieved between the stick's free end and the object. In a particularly apposite phrase, Piaget says that up to this point in time (about the first birthday) the child has commanded nature; from now on he does so by obeying it.

The foundation for the child's understanding of the nature of cause and effect relationships is securely laid when he is able to work out the cause of something happening without having seen the cause actually in operation. Thus at 18 months a variety of events which have been induced by the parents' actions are unhesitatingly attributed to them despite their having taken the utmost trouble to avoid letting the child see what they are doing. Evidence can be found of this occurring earlier; a child in his pram suddenly feels it being rocked without anyone holding it and he promptly leans over the side and smiles when he sees his father's foot moving the pram, as if he knew that there must be some cause and has now found it. The child realizes the necessity for a cause, and is becoming able to reconstruct or represent it in his mind from the effects it produces even when it is invisible. The same thing happens the other way round, and the child is beginning to be able to anticipate certain effects from certain actions he makes. At this age many examples of behaviours persist from an earlier stage, in which the child seems to expect (or perhaps it is now only that he hopes) that an action of his such as hand waving, or vocalizing, or nodding his head will be effective in making the desired result come about.

With the stage of representation, which is achieved before the second birthday, it becomes possible for the child to develop an objective view of the universe which is pervaded by a lasting system of permanent objects and causal connections, ordered and rule-governed, and one in which the element of magic is disappearing. That it never does so for some people is an interesting regression, sometimes charming, sometimes harmful, depending on the circumstances and the personalities of those concerned. From now on, and for the first time, the child is able to place himself properly in his surroundings as an object. He begins to see himself as an element which is at times effective, acting casually, but also aware that he is one cause among many, with many agents acting on him, in space which exists regardless of him, everywhere transcending him.

The Nature of the Child's Environment

One of the characteristic ways we have of looking at the world is analytical, dividing it into categories so that what is put into one cannot be put into the other. Analysis is refined by creating a whole hierarchy of categories by this process of dichotomy, splitting the material to be studied into contrasting pairs with progressive narrowing and precision of definition of what it is we are studying. We might choose for instance to describe our environment somewhat austerely as being divided into two main components, animate and inanimate—the world of living creatures and the physical world of the basic substances and features of our planet and its climate. The world of the biologist is separated from and contrasted with the world of the geologist, the physicist and the astronomer. As is often the case this is both helpful and misleading. At first sight the immediate environment of the child could well be classified in such a way, with his family providing the living element and the features and objects of his home surroundings providing the inanimate elements of walls, doors, chairs and tables, cups, spoons and so on. Indeed, such an approach has provided the basis for discussion till now. But the great majority of the elements comprising the child's environment are themselves manmade, artefacts of our culture, and cannot have any meaning apart from we who use them. This is a distinctive feature of the human community, setting it apart from almost all other animal organizations with the exception of certain highly structured insect environments such as the nests of bees or termite hills far removed in evolutionary time, and to a lesser extent the constructions, notably of birds, which play a special part in the breeding and care of the young.

Bruner (1974) has emphasized how man lives in an increasingly manmade environment, and certainly in more highly specialized and city-dwelling communities the natural world is removed some distance from the child. The human environment is highly artefactual, and mankind is ceaselessly active in adapting the natural world, processing and reconstructing it to suit human requirements. There is in this a cultural equivalent to the young child's encounters with his environment. As he receives and processes sensory information, actively meeting the world head- (and hand-) on, he reconstructs it internally within the neuropsychological processes of his central nervous system. The human child has a vast amount of learning to do in order to equip himself for living effectively within this man-made world, which has been developing the intricacy of its structures during presumably some few millions of years. This is over above and in addition to the progressive acquaintance and experience of its world required of every animal who is to survive until it is at the appropriate level of maturity to reproduce its kind.

If the child is to acquire the ability to live in the immensely complex system we call human society with its unending array of physical artefacts of all shapes, purposes and sizes, and the even more bewildering array of social customs, attitudes, and rule-governed behaviour which regulate personal and group interaction, then he must be equipped with highly effective tools which will enable him to learn about it and participate in it. These tools, which enable him to shape his own behaviour and gain some mastery of his environment, are the cognitive processes of imitation, play and above all, of language. Language is dependent upon imitation and play and the cognitive processes which underlie them, and without them cannot develop. Both these processes need therefore to be considered before the early stages of language development can be discussed.

Imitation

The fundamental importance of imitation is seen clearly in the progressive elaboration and shaping of the young child's vocalization. Through its influence his non-verbal utterances approximate more and more closely to the sound patterns of the adults and other children around him as they speak. Imitation takes other forms and is not confined to hearing and vocalization. Bower (1977) lists several ways in which the child less than a week old will copy what his mother is doing. He will, usually after some little delay, protrude his tongue in response to his mother putting hers out at him; similarly he will flutter his eyelashes or open and close his mouth. To this we must add evidence which suggests that vocal imitation may also occur in the first few days of life (see Chapter 4). These are all actions he carries out spontaneously but because of the appearance of the activity soon after the model provided by his mother, it is difficult to escape the conclusion that on these occasions he is imitating her.

The development of imitation has been studied systematically by Piaget. In "Play, Dreams and Imitations" (1962) he provides many valuable insights into its nature and functions, and it is to his work therefore that we turn once again for a description of the process, and to gain some understanding of its purpose. In the early months there is no ability to imitate what is new as far as the actions for the child are concerned; he imitates the movements and actions of others which he is already able to perform. Even here he will run into difficulties if he tries to carry out what might be called a sub-routine, a component of a larger action, however much he uses it in the course of the larger action. He is able to reach out and take hold of an object at six months, but is unable to imitate the more limited action of opening and closing his hand. Two or three months later the child is beginning to be able to imitate movements which are not visible to him when he in his turn attempts to copy them. In the case of one of his children Piaget found that she was not able to copy him when he put his tongue out at her at 8 months, and only succeeded in doing so nearly six weeks later having gone through a series of movements of the mouth, tongue and lips in which she made the attempt but failed to copy the model.

This failure of imitation contrasts so vividly with the observations made on the child in the first week of life, which Piaget does not seem to have observed, that one must ask if both processes can be called imitation. The basic facts seem to be the same—the child is presented with a model, in this case an adult putting out her tongue, which is copied successfully at one week and at nine months or so. But there has been an intervening period in which the task has been quite beyond the voluntary control of the child to imitate. One is obliged to conclude that though stimulus and response appear to be the same at the two ages the underlying mechanism are very different, requiring in the older child the elaboration and functioning of neurological pathways which are not available to the neonate. This need not cause too much difficulty if it is remembered that certain other motor behaviours develop in essentially the same way. The neonate for instance, if he is held firmly under the arms in the upright position so that his feet are in contact with a couch or table-top, will show alternating movements of his legs akin to walking. This primary form of walking is clearly very different from that seen in the child as he begins to walk round the room supported by one of his parents or the furniture he clings on to. The progressive development of central nervous structures, and their coming on-line in the organization and control of movement patterns is seen in other forms of imitation. From very early on the child has been able to put his finger in his mouth and suck it, but may not be able to carry out the deliberate imitation of his mother as she does it in front of him until 9 months. Opening and closing the eyes may lead the child to open and close his mouth in erroneous imitation until able to copy successfully, using movements of his own he cannot see, which may not be until he is a year old.

From the end of the first year the child is able to establish the correspondence between the parts of other people's faces and his own eyes and ears, nose, mouth and cheeks, shown by touching or patting them with his hand. This stage is important because of the implications it carries for other types of imitation;

"This study of imitation reveals the striking fact that when the child becomes capable of imitating movements he has already made, but which he cannot see on his own body, he also tries to copy sounds and gestures that are new to him, and which hitherto left him indifferent." (Piaget, 1962, p. 45)

Sounds and movements which are new now seem to be particularly attractive models for him to copy and give rise to immediate attempts at reproduction. From about the time of his first birthday he is able to imitate actions in which he cannot see the parts of his body he is using for his own activity in copying, and he is able to copy actions which he himself has not used before. The relevance of this newly attained level of skill for hearing and verbal utterances will be considered later. In the field of vision and motor activity it means that the child will for instance try to copy her father when he touches the tip of his tongue with his finger. This is copied immediately, but inaccurately. The child first touches her lip, then puts out her tongue without moving her finger, and then finally succeeds, by feeling for her tongue and touching its tip. Imitation has become more flexible and at the same time more experimental and persevering. Once the child is able to copy movements using activity which he cannot control visually, the next stage of abstraction is reached in which the model is not copied there and then, but at some later time. This means that it is no longer necessary for the child to see (or to hear) the model, but this can be represented or imaged and stored internally for use later. When Piaget's elder daughter was 16 months old she saw a familiar visitor, a boy two months older, get into a temper, stamping his feet and trying to get out of the playpen. This was a new experience for her and she watched in amazement; the next day she herself screamed in her playpen and stamped her foot in clear imitation of what she had seen. Her younger sister when she had reached the same age copied a characteristic habit of the older one precisely, rolling up a towel into a ball, drying her mouth with it, and then tucking it under her chin, though her sister was not present that particular bathtime.

It seems likely that these more complex and advanced forms of imitation have a well-developed cognitive basis, and that there is purpose in them. At this same age the younger sister was trying vainly to get a watch chain out of a matchbox which was only very slightly open. She gazed intently at the box and began to open and close her mouth, first only slightly, then wider and wider. This would appear to be an effort of the child to picture the event, representing it to herself so that she could then take the appropriate and effective action. From the description given it would seem to be a very clear example of non-verbal behaviour portraying and so revealing her thinking as she tries to understand the problem and reach a solution. It may be that the activity contained in the mental image she was using and operating on became more clearly defined in her mind as she imitated an opening and closing action with which she was already very familiar. This internal reproduction of the activity (which in other instances might instead be an object) is the beginning of symbol formation, and reveals the important part which imitation has to play in the process. Imitation should be looked upon as a continuation of the attempt to grasp the meaning of a situation or event; it is a part of the process of understanding, using internalized images or symbols, and not an end in itself. This is not possible until the child has reached the stage when he can store and retain images internally and subsequently reproduce them, as is shown for instance by deferred imitation.

"Since the imitation is already 'deferred', it implies the image, but in our view the image consists of interiorized imitation. Now, however, the image acquires a life of its own, and the child who imitates is often unaware that he is doing so. His response to the model seems to him to come from within himself, which means that his imitation is a continuation of his interior images and not that it gives rise to them." (Piaget, 1962, pp. 74 and 75)

This must surely not only be true for the child but for all of us. A particularly striking personal example in which it is possible to date the temporal relationships quite accurately relates to a drawing I was asked to make on the spur of the moment by my wife when she was preparing a lesson for young Sunday School children. I drew a large picture of Solomon's Temple in Jerusalem, relying so I thought on knowledge of the description in the First Book of Kings, chapters 6 and 7. It was not until some years later that realization dawned. My highly original drawing was an almost perfect replica in perspective and orientation, and in the details of its plinth, steps, pillars and side buildings, of an illustration in Grollenberg (1959) which I had not looked at for 2–3 years previous to making the drawing. This singular example of remarkably precise imitation deferred over years, with no conscious recollection of the model being copied, reveals the power of imitation, and it is more prevalent in our lives than we might sometimes choose to imagine. Some of our most original and innovative thoughts have the same antecedents as my drawing, previous experiences and perceptions simply awaiting the time and the place to be reproduced.

Play

Play is a widespread feature of animal life and is especially characteristic of the young human; not only this but adult humans participate in many forms of games and resort to subtle forms of play, verbal and otherwise whenever the opportunity presents and not infrequently when it has not presented. The effects of teasing, and the embarrassed or baffled responses to inopportune play of this sort are often sufficient reward in themselves. Clinical experience reveals that play is an essential precursor to language and the child who shows impairment of his ability to play almost always has difficulty in learning to talk, when compared with his normally developing peers. The converse is by no means always true, and many children with severe language deficits can show an advanced and imaginative level of play. When one pauses to consider the numerous forms of activity all subsumed under the one word "play" it will be appreciated that the verbal concept is far too diffuse to be of any practical or theoretical value without careful description of what is under discussion. We should talk, not so much about play, as about specific play activities or behaviours.

If simple repetitive activity, carried on apparently with no other purpose than for the sake of the activity itself, is accompanied by evidence of pleasure shown by smiling, or a little later by laughter, then play can be said to occur during or soon after the second month. It may be manifested in patterns of vocalization, or in the fixing and deliberate severing of gaze playfully repeated, or in other movements of the head or hands. As the child gains further control of his activity, the serious attempts by which he learns to carry out particular actions become transformed into playful repetitions once he has mastered them, and they are then performed for the pure pleasure of doing them, with no other apparent purpose. With increasing sensorimotor proficiency the child will not simply repeat one particular action or behaviour, but will combine it with another, or several others in a sequence. Later these sequences are combined in a less random and more formalized way and become rituals. It is instructive to look at the observations recorded by Piaget on the developing play behaviours shown by his daughter, Jacqueline, in relation to going to sleep. When she was just 9 months old she carried out a whole series of playful activities with the toys and other objects in her cot ending up with taking hold of her pillow and shaking it about.

"As she was holding the pillow, she noticed the fringe, which she began to suck. This action, which reminded her of what she did every day before going to sleep, caused her to lie down on her side, in the position for sleep, holding a corner of the fringe and sucking her thumb. This, however, did not last for half a minute, and Jacqueline resumed her earlier activity." (Piaget, 1962, p. 93)

The ritual is in effect a programme of activities combined together into a sequence—sucking the fringe, lying down, turning on her side, holding the fringe, sucking her thumb, closing her eyes. Later these rituals become more and more involved, as anyone will recall who has been driven to distraction by a child at a later age preparing to go to bed. We need to be tolerant of these rituals because we all show evidence of them, whether it be the protracted preparations some people go through before they actually start eating the food on their plates; the various rituals which must be completed before or at the end of a sporting event such as a game of football or horse racing; or the splendour and sophistication of some State ceremonial.

Some childhood rituals are initiated accidentally, as when Piaget's Jacqueline, shortly after her first birthday, was grasping her hair with her hand which then slipped and struck the water with a splash. Once she had worked out and successfully imitated what she had done, this action was carried out with the regularity of a ritual every bath-time for a while. A similar example seen in the clinic concerned a two-year-old boy who accidentally fell off his chair onto the floor, and promptly repeated the activity four or five times more until he chanced to knock his leg against the table and was reduced to tears. There is no purpose behind such activities, which seem on the contrary to be carried out purely for the pleasure the child derives from them, and as the child increases in age so he deliberately increases the complexity of the sequence. These rituals are important in that they provide the basis for the transition to symbolic play in which true pretend and make-believe appear. This change takes place at about the time when the child is able to store the images he is imitating and reproduce them later, when he chooses. When Jacqueline was three months older than at the time of the "going-to-sleep" ritual she showed the first evidence of make-believe play.

"She saw a cloth whose fringed edges vaguely recalled those of her pillow; she seized it, held a fold of it in her right hand, sucked the thumb of the same hand and lay down on her side, laughing hard. She kept her eyes open, but blinked from time to time as if she were alluding to closed eyes." (Piaget, 1962, p. 96)

In the next days and weeks the game was initiated with objects which were less and less like the original fringed edge of her pillow, and the element of pretend becomes progressively more evident. By 17 months she was not carrying out the action for herself but instead was making her toy animals do it. Within the next two or three months she carried out a number of pretend activities, such as washing her hands or eating various things when there was nothing there, or the article was only nominally represented. The symbolic activity arises frequently out of the progressive abstraction of the preceding patterns of ritual, until it is no longer necessary for the object to be physically represented, since it is represented internally in the child's imagination. The image can then be used by the child at will, and he seems to derive particular pleasure from distorting reality and so, as it were, playing with it.

The process of imitation remains an essential element in the elaboration of play activities. From the brief imitation of simple domestic activities at 18 months, pretending to feed a doll or read a book or sweep the floor, the child progresses to more elaborate pretend play with doll's prams, and the larger representational toys, and will follow his mother around the house as she makes the beds, dusts and sweeps, and does the washing up, imitating her activities (Sheridan, 1975; 1977). This imitative early role play becomes progressively more inventive; the child imagines himself to be engaged in a wide range of roles and pursuits, and is subsequently able to fabricate the necessary stage props out of what comes to hand. Before this highly developed play has appeared there has been a similar progression in the way the child comes to understand the significance of miniature play materials such as doll's-house-sized furniture. At 15 months such things are merely objects which have no representational quality, but are things to be put in and out of boxes or piled up one on top of the other. By 21 months the child is able to show by the way she arranges these objects that she has grasped the basic relations which exist between say a miniature table and chair and, soon after the second birthday, organizes the materials into a simple but effective replica of everyday reality. The same pattern of development is seen with other types of toy, such as the ever popular car, which is at first something simply to push backwards and forwards with no understanding of its significance, until at a later age the child is able to represent cars lined up on roads, backing and turning, filling up with petrol, making way for the ambulance and so on. Even without the accompaniment of words this type of play reveals very clearly how well the child is able to understand the meaning of the world around, and recreate it for himself in play.

4 Vocal Behaviour and the Origins of Speech

The Cry

The newborn child's first spontaneous behaviour is heard rather than seen, and the cry is eagerly awaited as an indicator of the onset of normal respiration and of independent existence. Once established the cry is such a commonplace behaviour it is easily dismissed as being unimportant, and not worthy of serious study. It has however attracted a certain amount of interest by for instance Lynip (1951) and Eisenson, Auer, and Irwin (1963). Wasz-Höckert and his colleagues (1968) have also studied the features of the cry in certain disorders such as brain-damage at birth, and chromosomal abnormalities resulting in particular clinical states such as the "cri du chat" syndrome. Wolff (1969) studied the cry of children during the first six months of life, motivated by his interest in the development of the various forms of human affective expression. He identified four main types of cry. The most frequently occurring "basic" cry has a predominant fundamental frequency of 350—400 Hz and is often called the hunger cry, though Wolff considers that this term is misleading if it is used to imply a causal connection between hunger and a particular pattern of crying. Other cries are the "mad" or angry cry, and the cry caused by pain. This latter is characterized by a sudden onset of loud crying without any preliminary fussing, an initial long cry lasting 3—4 seconds, and a subsequent long period of breath-holding in the expiratory phase before the next cry. He concluded that "the range of causal conditions sufficient to provoke crying in the neonate is greater than has been taken for granted, and that very early in development the infant cries in response to environmental conditions which should be viewed as having a global *psychological* significance since they cannot be analyzed in physical—physiological terms alone" (Wolff, 1969, p. 108, his italics). Muller, Hollien, and Murry (1974) in a follow-up study of earlier work carried out by Wasz-Höckert, Partanen *et al.*, (1964) found that mothers of young children were not able to identify specific features of tape-recorded cries which would enable them to distinguish between pain, loud auditory stimulation or startle, and hunger as the determinant of the onset of the cry. This was true whether the mother was listening to her own or the other infants in the series, all tending to over-interpret the cries as due to hunger. They had very little difficulty in recognizing which cries were produced by their own child. In a later study, Murry, Amundson, and Hollien (1977) found that the mean fundamental frequency of the hunger cry was 438.5 Hz, of the pain cry 441 Hz and of the startle cry 421.3 Hz, for four boys and four girls aged 3—6 months. From the data as reported one may calculate the standard deviation (SD) of the cry frequency; this is ± 48.4 Hz for the hunger cry, and clearly the perceived pitch of a sequence of cries cannot help the listener determine the reason for the cry. This is amply confirmed by the results of other investigations of the frequency of the cry. Wasz-Höckert, Lind *et al.* (1968) found the mean to be 530 Hz for pain (SD 80 Hz) and 500 Hz for hunger cries (SD 70 Hz) during the period from 1—7 months old.

There is a notable tendency to interpret cries and all the child's earlier vocalization as being due to one of a small range of causes, including hunger, pain, comfort and discomfort. This approach overlooks the possibility that such terms may not have the meaning for the infant which they hold for the adult observer. We need a great deal more information on the structure and sequential arrangement of cries and other non-linguistic vocal behaviours before turning to the "semantics" or significance of such behaviours.

The duration of the sound of each individual cry shows considerable variation, as may be seen in Fig. 4.1 a. The histogram represents the cries of seven children, boy and girl, African and English, aged 0—41 days, without regard to the type of cry. The

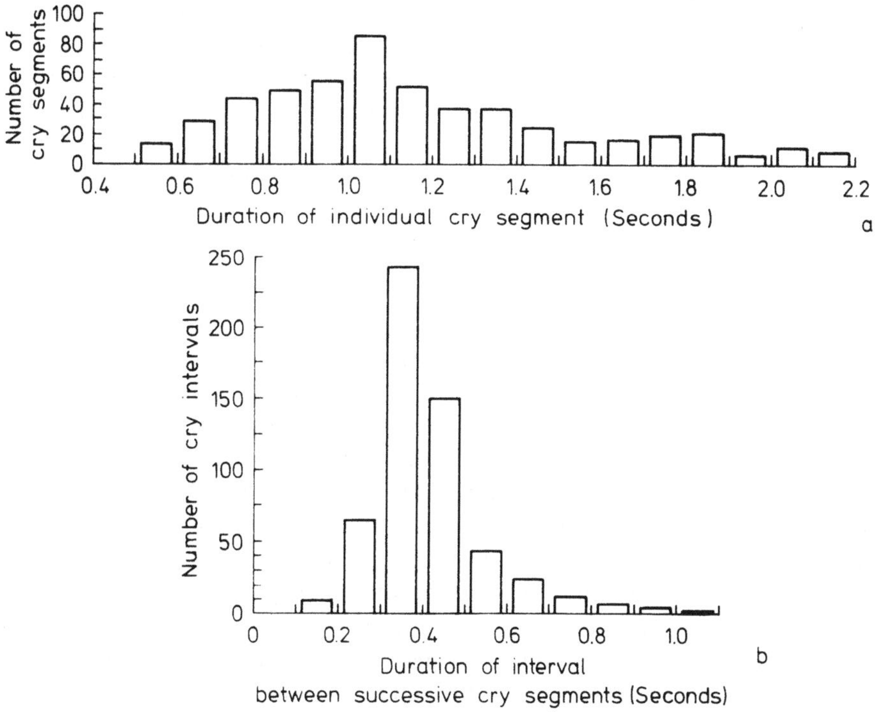

Fig. 4.1. *a* Duration of cry segments for seven children 0—41 days, *b* Inter-cry duration for seven children aged 0—41 days

mean duration of the sound segment is 0.89 sec (SD 0.52 sec). If one looks at the interval between two adjacent cries there is a much higher degree of uniformity for its duration (Fig. 4.1 b), the mean being 0.43 sec (SD 0.21 sec). These two values combined give a cry rate averaging 46 cry segments a minute. If one looks at the same features at different ages no real differences emerge (Table 4.1) for the duration of the cry, and none at all for the intercry duration. It is difficult to escape the conclusion that the temporal characteristics of crying are innate and arise from the mechanical features of the respiratory tract, the chemical changes taking place in the circulating blood and pulmonary alveoli and rhythmical vocal patterning organized at a neurological level.

Table 4.1. *Duration of cry segment during first six weeks of life for three different age groups*

	0–6 days	7–27 days	28–41 days
Number of cries	150	371	76
Mean duration (seconds)	0.9 sec	0.85 sec	0.94 sec
Standard deviation	0.48	0.50	0.70

Early Vocal Behaviour

Several stages in the development of the vocal behaviour of young children have been identified and labelled; these include cooing, babbling and jargon and they are described as following on one from the other. The terms are used imprecisely and there is little agreement on the characteristics and age of appearance or the duration of these behaviours. They are in fact highly impressionistic terms which oversimplify the picture and turn the observer's attention away from numerous important sound-producing activities. In order to identify these various patterns and types of vocalization a series of time-sections will be examined, starting at the first day after birth. The first six weeks are represented by a number of sections, after which they are spaced at 4–6 week intervals.

Terminology

Before looking into the details of the time-sections it is necessary to consider an important general problem which arises out of terminology. Crystal (1973, 1975) in his review of non-segmental phonology in language acquisition has commented on the inconsistencies of nomenclature and the discrepancies which abound in the literature. The lack of specific terms is probably an indication of the lack of detailed exploration of early vocal behaviour, and from the understandable but largely unquestioned assumption that such behaviour is inevitably linguistic. It is preferable to explore the prelinguistic behaviour of children as a behaviour in its own right. The first step in this direction is to avoid the anticipatory term "prelinguistic", and refer instead to the child's vocal activity, which is used here to refer to any sound-producing behaviour of the child before specifically linguistic items can be identified. This end-point is itself extremely difficult to identify, and each of us will differ over what is meant. There are features characteristic of language which occur early on in the first year such as certain vowel and consonant sounds or intonation patterns. If these are heard is it not reasonable to say that the child is using linguistic elements? Looking at the question from a functional aspect, one might say that attempts to produce sounds which might be interpreted in any way as purposeful or communicative, and to which the mother might be able to attribute "meaning" are examples of linguistic usage. Whilst not denying the value of such arguments, it may be said that they do nothing to help avoid confusion in the minds of the non-cognoscenti. Spoken "language" as used here is consistent with the definition in Webster (1971): "the words, their pronounciation, and the methods of combining them used and understood by a considerable community and established by long usage". Even if the "considerable community" is reduced to the child's mother and perhaps his father and siblings for a few short weeks we will adhere to a common-sense definition of "words", and look upon their appearance as heralding the beginnings of language as such. Until this stage is reached, usually shortly after the first birthday, it is essential to avoid the use of terms which have a linguistic connotation. Rather than list them here, appropriate words will be introduced and defined in context as the necessity arises.

The Recorded Material

In the pages which follow, the child's personal name, ethnic origin, sex and age are given. No two children have the same name. The convention has been adopted that the age is shown in months (M) and decimals of a month, calculated from the basis that there are 30.4 days in a calendar month. One decimal point (0.1 M) may be taken as representing 3 days. This convention has been used because it is an appropriate time span in which to note changing patterns of vocal behaviour, it avoids an over-detailed and somewhat cumbrous approach inherent in reports in which the number of days is stated, and calculation is greatly facilitated should it be required. The figures are all taken from the trace of a Bruel and Kjaer sound level recorder with the paper speed running at 10 mm per sec. and the writing speed of the pen set at 100 mm per sec. In order to accommodate these figures on the printed page there has been a reduction in size so that each second of duration is represented by fractionally over 5 mm down the length of the page. All the tape-recordings illustrated, and indeed all the recordings of the children's vocal activity from which the figures in this chapter have been selected as representative of that particular age, were analyzed initially by transcribing them at a paper transport speed of 30 mm per sec, and a pen writing speed of 250 mm per sec.

The full body of recorded material relates to 23 children, 12 girls and 11 boys; 14 of them were English, 7 were from the three countries of East Africa (Uganda, Kenya and Tanzania) exposed almost entirely to their own tribal language, and 2 were of Indian origin though born in Kampala. The recordings were made as frequently as possible, usually weekly or fortnightly, and starting as soon after birth as could be arranged. They were recorded on a variety of models of recording equipment often under somewhat adverse circumstances over a number of years. It was possible to continue recording 7 children after their first six months of life, this number decreasing to 4 (an African and an English child of either sex) by 12 months, and an unrelated English boy and girl were followed up for two years from birth.

Chronological Sections of Vocal Behaviour

1. Peter; English, boy 22 hours

The basic features of the cry have already been discussed. Fig. 4.2* represents the vocal activity of a newly born child just after he has been replaced in his cot after being fed. He was not crying but was simply engaged in spontaneous sound production. The sounds are brief, with a mean duration of 0.45 sec but they show a surprising degree of variation in loudness, in pitch and voice quality, in duration and in patterning. It is not possible to quantify loudness levels because of variation from one recording session to another, background noise and activity (over which one may have to accept no control is possible) and the movements of the child as he turns his head towards and away from the microphone. It is possible to gain in idea of the relative loudness of successive vocalizations by estimating the height or (with the vertical orientation of the trace adopted here) the distance of the peak from the baseline on the left hand margin. The pitch varies from 260 Hz, when the voice is low and creaky, through a well modulated middle range of the order of 360—420 Hz, to a thin high-pitched fundamental laryngeal frequency of up to 660 Hz. The sound is perceived by an adult English speaker as predominantly /ə/ or "er". The sounds are not restricted to being vowel-like in quality; 7 out of the 19 vocalizations (V) 2, 3, 5, 6, 8, 19 and 20 start with a distinct "h" consonant quality. The sounds may be single with only one pulse of sound to the vocalization, or the child may continue breathing out and produce a second pulse of sound, perceived as a definite "er" but not entirely separate from the first. This is most clearly seen in V.1, V.13, V.14, and in these vocalizations the duration may be from 0.7 sec to as long as 1.73 sec.

The problem of nomenclature already arises. Reference has perforce been made to vowel and consonant sounds. These are terms which can only be used within a linguistic frame of reference. The convention will be adopted that in the weeks and months before words can be identified, but at a time when the child is producing vowel-like and consonant-like sounds these will be termed *vowelals* and *consonantals* and represented by the phonetic character which approximates most closely to the sound but enclosed in square brackets, *e.g.* [bə] or "ber". At an earlier stage still, during the first few months of life, the vowel-like and consonant-like sounds are usually so far removed from normal speech that even this convention is

---

* In this and the illustrations of vocal behaviour which follow, the columns represent (from left to right):

(1) The visual display of the Brüel & Kjaer sound-level recorder, type 2305; the continous line indicates the variations in intensity of the tape-recorded signal.

(2) The sequential number of the child's vocalization.

(3) A transcription of the sound value of the vocal (or later verbal) utterance of the child, using as far as practicable the symbols of the International Phonetic Alphabet. ***An explanation of the symbols used and an indication of their sound values is given on pp. XIV—XVI.***

(4) The consecutive utterances of the mother *(M)*, father *(F)*, recordist *(R)* etc. Adventitious noises which may cause confusion are indicated eg. car noise.

(5) The time in seconds, marked also on the trace of the sound-level recorder.

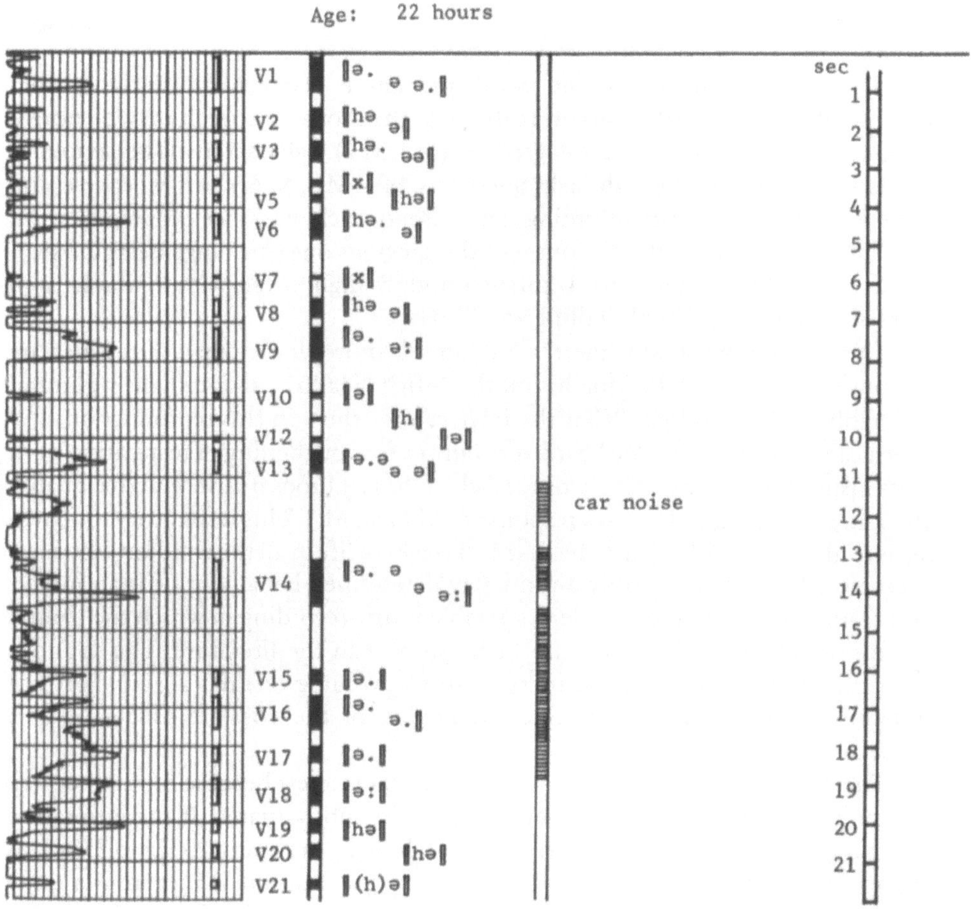

Fig. 4.2

misleading. We will label these sounds *vocants* and *closants* and their transcription will be enclosed within double square brackets *e.g.* [[bə]]. This emphasizes the remoteness of the sounds from ordinary speech sounds, and though the phonetic characters used are intended to convey something of the perceived quality of the vocalization, it should not be assumed even that the infant is making the sound in the same way that the linguistically competent speaker does.

We are obliged to conclude that the newborn child is capable of spontaneous, surprisingly well-controlled vocalization in which the antecedents of syllabic patterning may already be apparent. It is not possible to accept that these vocalizations should be classed either as discomfort or as comfort sounds. They are neither, but instead have a curiously purposeful, definite quality, faint though some of them are. The most appropriate analogy may be with that of the movements of a newborn foal, struggling to its kness and onto its feet and taking its first collapsing steps. There is a necessity about this activity, ordained as it is by the animal's innate neurology, and the vocalization of the human newborn has the same quality.

2. Peter 2 days

Fig. 4.3 shows the nature of the vocal interaction between mother and child which is already apparent. Certain features of the mother's speech may be noted; she greets her child and repeats her greeting (M.1, M.2), a characteristic behaviour of adults with young children; she asks questions, M.3, M.4, M.6; she is repetitive, and there is a certain regularity of timing. The onset of each utterance occurs at a mean time interval of 2.3 sec after the onset of the previous one (the range being 1.8 sec—2.9 sec, SD 0.4 sec). Her voice is pitched unduly high, often with a simple, well marked cadence, *e.g.* 510 Hz falling to 275 Hz.

The child is not listening inertly, but himself shows vocal behaviours which are responsive in nature. Following his mother's first "Hallo" a small, slightly guttural "(h)erghh" (V.1) is uttered. What the trace cannot show in this reproduction, and which can in any case only be heard very faintly, is a roughening of respiration both in its inspiratory and expiratory phases which has a purposeful, interactive quality about it. It may be seen here as a response to M.1 and M.3. This respiratory roughening is readily detectable within the first 2—3 weeks of life in all the children who have been recorded and is probably an innately determined behaviour. It is an important feature of interaction, not demonstrable in any recording in which the child is left to himself, and yet there is no mention of it in the literature. The sound is probably produced through an increase in the volume of tidal air and force of respiration, and by partial sustained adduction of the vocal folds during 2—5 consecutive breaths.

There is another vocal behaviour of particular interest because of the theoretical implications it raises if the observation can be substantiated. If the intonation contour of the mother's "Happy boy" (M.5), falling from about 420 Hz to 250 Hz is compared with the pitch contour of the child's vocalization V.5, there is a quite remarkable similarity of tonal change over time (Fig. 4.4). The likelihood that the utterances of the mother and the child are related is increased by the vocal behaviour V.4. There are two distinct roughened respirations; these are often found to lead into a more explicit vocalization as if they were the preparatory phase of it. His mother follows on with M.6 which is a question and has a different tonal pattern from M.5 and then the child's vocalization is released, almost as if it had been temporarily inhibited by her utterance. Bearing in mind the imitation and interaction demonstrated by Condon and Sanders (1974) at the same age it is reasonable to suppose that this child is carrying out the vocal equivalent of interactional synchrony.

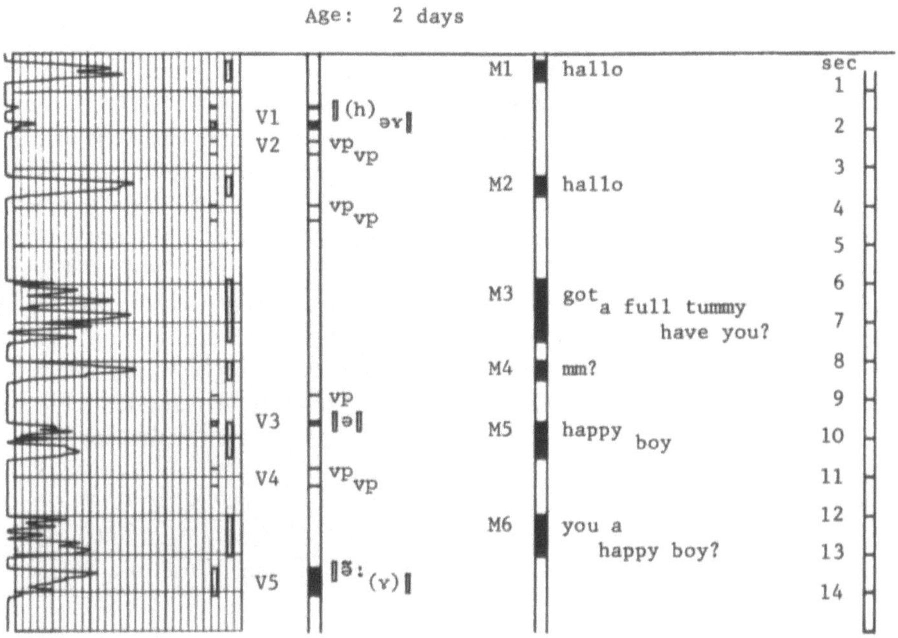

Fig. 4.3

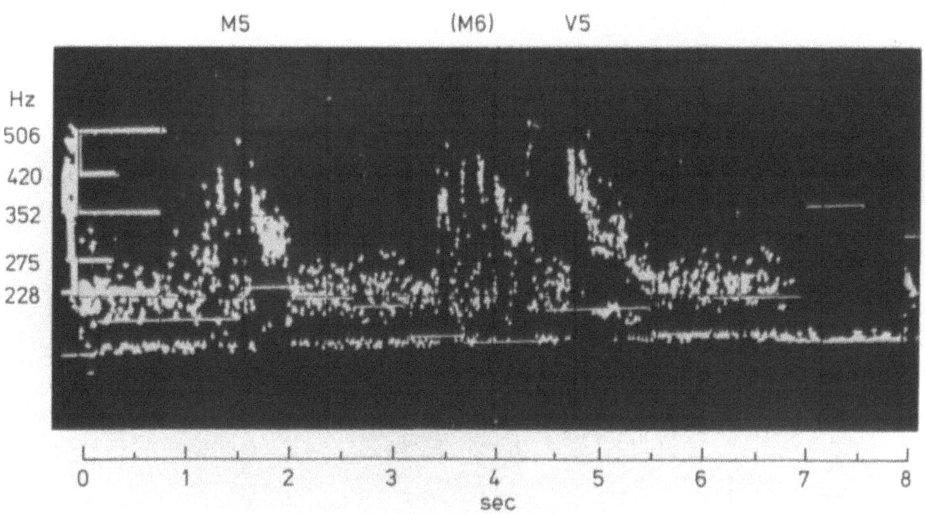

Fig. 4.4. Vocal pitch. Child 2 days old; showing close similarity between vocal pitch changes of second half of mother's utterance M.5, "(happy) boy" and child's vocal response V.5. The utterance M.6 should probably be disregarded (see text). This and subsequent illustrations of pitch contours are photographs of the long-persist oscilloscope screen of the "Visipitch" equipment. The utterances may be identified from the analysis of the tape-recorded material using the sound-level recording which accompanies each time section

3. Peter 3 days

Fig. 4.5 shows a series of vocalizations which increase in loudness and vehemence until cries are produced. The child is waiting for a feed. The first six vocalizations are short, with the exception of V.4 which is continued for just over 1 sec and has a second pulse of sound. More remarkable is the pattern of pitch change (Fig. 4.6). V.2 increases in fundamental frequency from 290 Hz to 370 Hz in less than 0.4 sec, V.3 shows a falling and rising pattern of pitch change, from 610 Hz down to 500 Hz and up again to 600 Hz in 0.23 sec, and V.6 shows the reverse pattern of rising and falling pitch, from 360 Hz up to a peak of 730 Hz and falling to 510 Hz in 0.17 sec. The first sound clearly identified as a cry shows a different pattern (V.13) and the two preceding sounds show a transitional appearance from the earlier brief pulses of vocant sound, with some elongation and holding of the vocalization at its loudest point. A cry segment tends to start moderately loud, increase in loudness to a peak and then fall quite rapidly, often with a sharp, brief ingressive terminal phase which may be separate from the cry sound as in V.13 and markedly so in V.16, or almost indistinguishable from it as in V.15. The pitch change in a cry segment is relatively slight, V.13 showing a rise from 310 Hz to 400 Hz and down again, and V.15 shows a continuous rise between the same two limits.

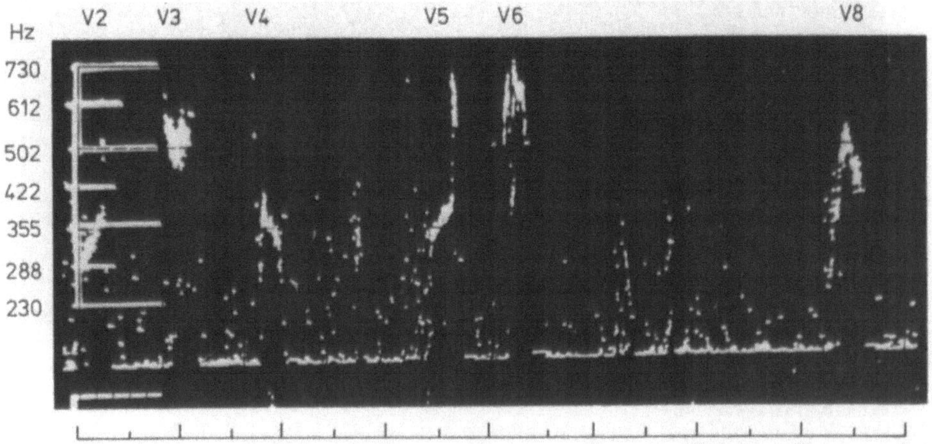

Fig. 4.6. Vocal pitch. Variety of patterns of pitch change produced by child 3 days old. The predominant pitch change seen here is a sharp rise-fall contour with a maximum height of approximately 390 Hz (V.4), 730 Hz (V.6) and 510 Hz (V.8). Other pitch contours may be identified

Age: 3 days

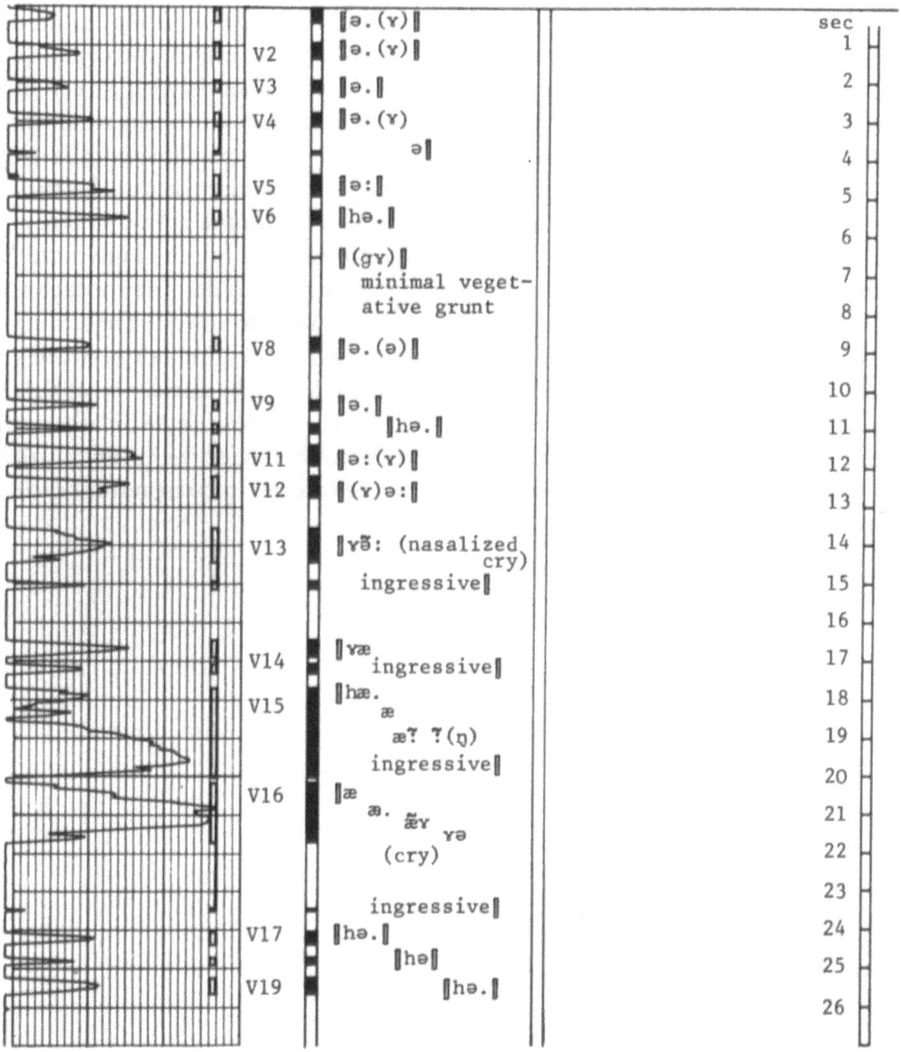

Fig. 4.5

4. Mary; Luhya, a Bantu tribe from Western Kenya, girl 5 days (0.2 M)

Fig. 4.7 shows a series of brief vocalizations and is interactive in nature though the father's voice cannot easily be demonstrated as it is restricted to very quiet soothing sounds. The child utters a number of vocant sounds with a very short single pulse lasting 0.1 sec and then suddenly at V.9 produces a vocalization which has no less than 4 pulses on a single breath in 1 sec. The next three vocalizations have two or three pulses until V.13 which repeats the four-pulse pattern, this time in 0.63 sec. The remaining sounds revert to a single pulse of sound, but now there is an increasing amount of closant sound, the child introducing a minimal unvoiced "h" at the beginning of V.16 which is rather more prolonged and definite for each subsequent sound until there is clear laryngeal friction audible at V.19. The timing of these latter sounds from V.14—19 is surprisingly regular, the intervals between successive onsets of sound being 0.65, 0.5, 0.6, 0.6 and 0.6 sec. She also shows at V.4 the panting, respiratory roughening previously referred to, three of these breaths occurring at one second intervals. In order to identify this behaviour in future it will be labelled a vocal pant (vp); each is a clearly audible exaggerated respiratory cycle of inspiration and expiration.

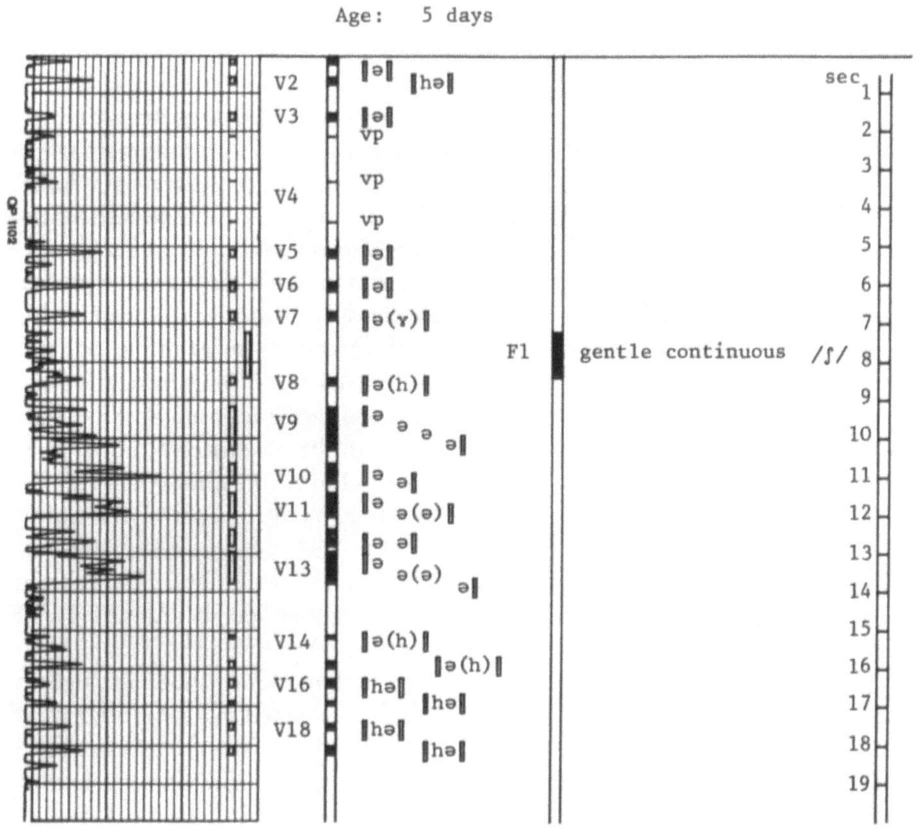
Age: 5 days
V2
V3
V4
V5
V6
V7
V8
V9
V10
V11
V13
V14
V16
V18
vp
vp
vp
F1
gentle continuous
/ʃ/
sec
1
2
3
4
5
6
7
8
9
10
11
12
13
14
15
16
17
18
19

Fig. 4.7

5. Stephen; English, boy 2 weeks (0.5 M)

He has just woken up, begins to make occasional very quiet sounds and these increase in number and loudness. By the beginning of Fig. 4.8 he is uttering strong brief pulses of vocant sound and cries then begin to appear. The temporal characteristics of V.1—8 are remarkably constant: the mean duration of the sounds is 0.11 sec with a deviation of 15 msec (0.015 sec), and the periodicity is 0.49 sec with a deviation of 27 msec. The stability of vocal timing mechanisms is clearly of a high order, especially since for these very brief sounds there is no additional constraint from the effects of progressive build-up of carbon dioxide, or shortage of oxygen which limits the length of a sustained vocalization. V.12 is such an example, in which sound production and expiration continue for virtually 2.5 sec before a breath is taken; physiological changes in the circulating blood and lung gases must inevitably modify and set limits on such activity. But this is not the case with such brief pulses of sound seen in the first part of the section, which must be almost entirely controlled by neural activity alone in the appropriate parts of the central nervous system.

It is not easy to identify the fundamental frequency of these very brief sounds; V.1—10 show very little difference, all lying between about 560 Hz and 620 Hz. The cry segments are predominantly in the region of 380—420 Hz.

This section, taken with previous ones, reveals that crying is not so straightforward an activity as it sounds. It is unusual to find it restricted to a long, unchanging sequence of cry segments, and non-cry vocal behaviour is mixed inextricably. Whilst crying is rarely if ever heard without these brief pulses of vocant sound, often with a distinct closant "h" sound initially, it has been seen that these sounds do occur in the absence of cry. They almost certainly comprise the vocal behaviour from which the sound carrier wave of speech is developed and elaborated prior to the appearance of spoken language.

At this point we might return briefly to consider the nature of crying. Without doubt young children cry when they are hungry, when they are startled, or when sudden abdominal colic or other pain is experienced. It has already been noted that mothers, more especially the less experienced, place an undue emphasis on hunger as the cause. It seems at least as probable that the crying of babies may frequently be attributed to the desire to restore that physical reality of contact with another human being, and especially their mother. Wolff (1969) noted, and this accords well with all parental experience, that picking the crying child up is consistently among the most effective ways of getting the child to stop crying. Contact is restored, but it is almost certainly more than physical contact which is important; the child is in communion once again with his mother, physically, emotionally, cognitively. If this is the case, the vocal behaviour demonstrated by Stephen in this section may be interpreted as an awareness of being solitary after he has become fully awake, which is expressed by the increasing agitation or vehemence of his repeated brief vocalizations, until crying supervenes. A great deal of crying is probably instrumental in nature, ensuring the appearance of another person, and especially the one with whom the bonds of attachment are being strongly formed. For the adult, infant cry-

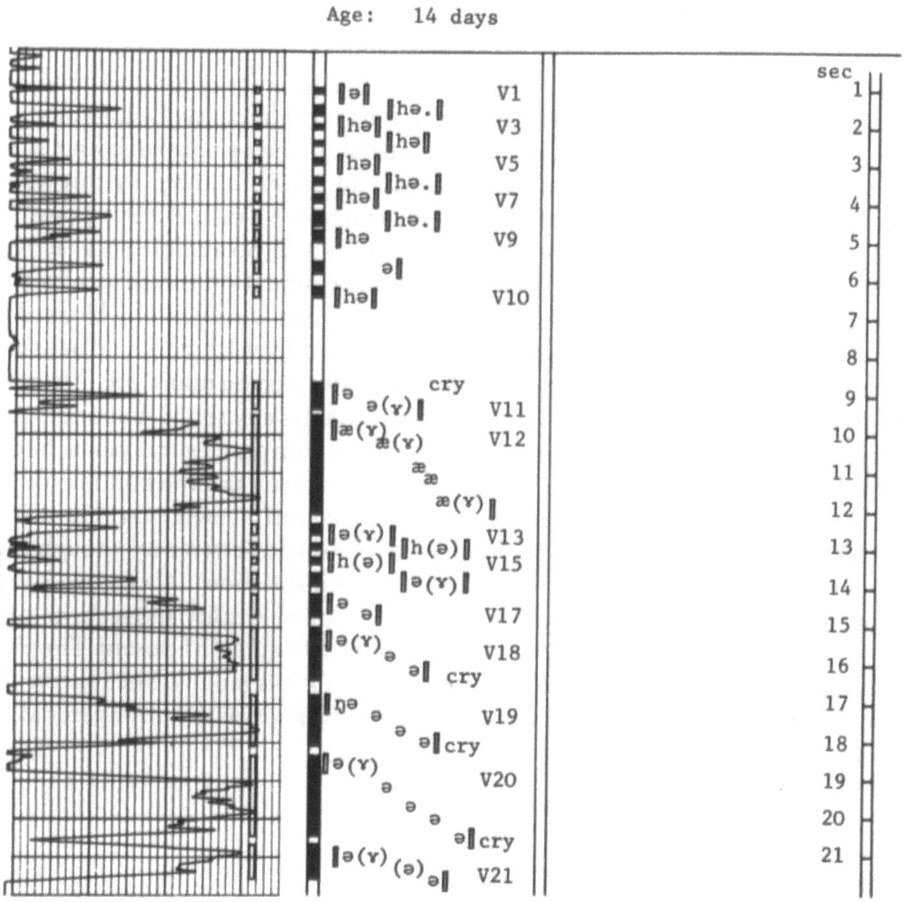

Fig. 4.8

ing is unsettling and difficult to ignore. It is therefore an important example of communitive behaviour and, in the first days and weeks, is one of the few behaviours the child has under his control.

6. Rosi; Lugbara, a Sudanic tribe from the extreme north-west of Uganda; girl 26 days (0.9 M)

Fig. 4.9 reveals a great deal of interaction taking place between the child and her father, who is able to modulate her behaviour very effectively by his voice, but she is far from being a passive partner. She starts by giving a single, unsustained cry which finishes with a sharp implosive sound, and this is followed by three brief vocal pulses, which is attenuated further to two vocal pants. At this point her father calls her name (F.1) and she stills completely, with no audible vocal activity until immediately after F.3. She begins to signal her intention to vocalize by four vocal pants which are produced in less than 1.5 sec; this is only briefly blocked by her father, and she utters a complex sound lasting just over 1.5 sec which has three separate pulses to it, the centre element sounding like a cry in miniature. After this effort she listens intently to F.5 with no attempt to utter any sound, but once again begins to signal her intention to vocalize after F.6 with three vocal pants. Something remarkable then happens. Her father remans silent and the build-up of her vocalization is able to continue free from distraction until it emerges as V.9 and V.10 (which should almost certainly be considered as a single "utterance" though they are separated by the implosive sound of a sharp inspiration). These two sound segments have a very gentle, carefully controlled singing quality about them, similar to a "coo" except that the "er" vocant is preceded by a quiet "h" closant. The pitch of each starts at 500 Hz and 560 Hz respectively and falls rapidly. She follows this effort with four strong vocal pants and a loud vocalization with a strong initial "h" closant sound and marked implosion after.

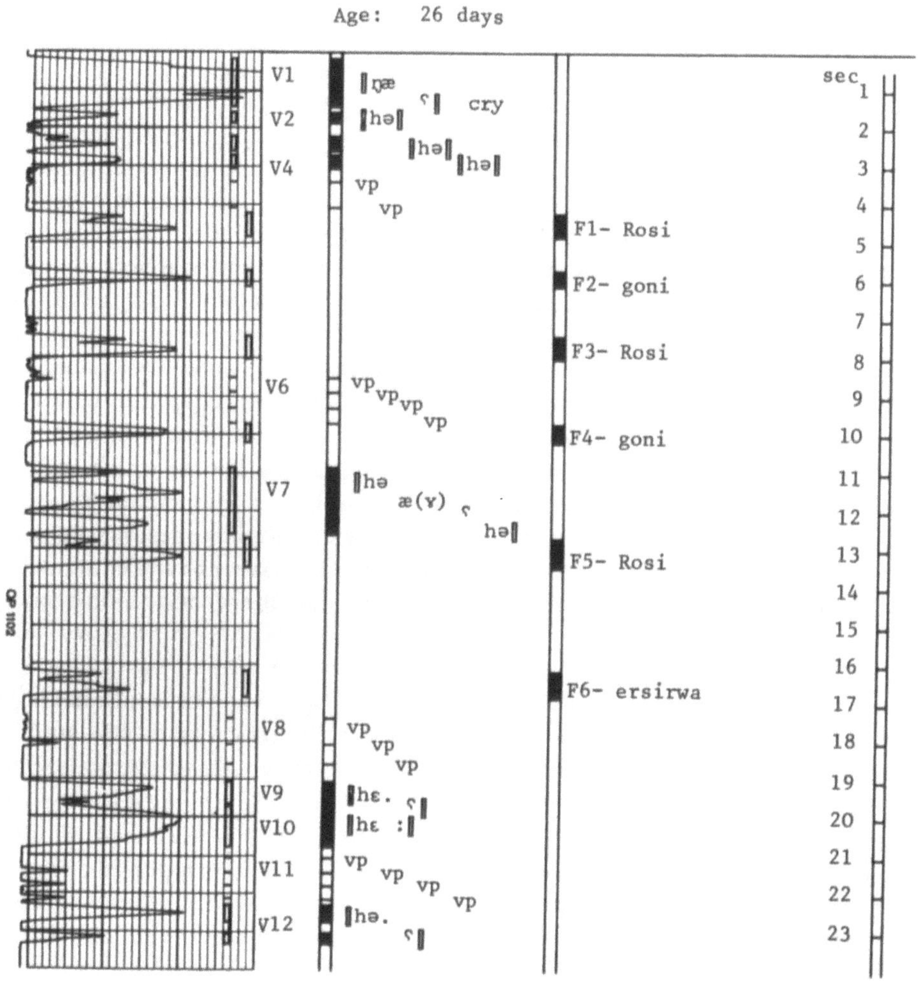
Age: 26 days
V1
V2
V4
V6
V7
V8
V9
V10
V11
V12
ŋæ ʕ cry
hə
hə hə
vp vp
vp vp vp vp
hə æ(ɤ) ʕ hə
vp vp vp
hɛ. ʕ
hɛ :
vp vp vp vp
hə. ʕ
F1- Rosi
F2- goni
F3- Rosi
F4- goni
F5- Rosi
F6- ersirwa
sec
1
2
3
4
5
6
7
8
9
10
11
12
13
14
15
16
17
18
19
20
21
22
23

Fig. 4.9

7. Peter 1.6 M

This interaction takes place halfway through a feed. His mother has taken him off the breast and the two are looking at each other when she says "Hallo Peter". Fig. 4.10 a starts 8.9 sec later, an interval during which neither of them makes another sound. The first six sounds which the child utters are single vocal pulses, each varying slightly from the previous one. This is followed by vocal panting (V.7) in which 6 pants occurred in 4.2 sec, a rate of 84 per min. This vocal behaviour is a marked feature of the recording, reappearing at V.9, V.12 and V.15, and taken with the other vocal activity gives a good indication of the intensity of the interaction from the child's side. The section takes the development shown in section 6 a stage further and the details are strikingly similar, apart from the mother spacing out her utterances more than Rosi's father. The particular feature to note takes place after M.3 (and compare this with the events in Section 6 after F.6). The child signals his intention to vocalize by vocal panting (V.15), there is an introductory trial vocalization and then a well-formed throaty vocant sound lasting 0.6 sec which ends in gentle pharyngeal friction. In less than a second the sound is repeated but the activity is speeded up a little and the closant sound is now followed by a separate pulse of vocant sound. This imparts a more specifically "g"-like quality to the closant and V.18 sounds like "ah(ger)" with two distinct pulses though the second is much quieter.

It might be thought that these two vocalizations are entirely fortuitous, but this would almost certainly prove to be erroneous. The interaction continues for a further 47 sec in a manner similar to the first part of the section up to V.16, with an occasional grunt, hiccup and other specifically "vegetative" sound also appearing. In Fig. 4.10 b however the child can be seen to reproduce his earlier more patterned vocalizations; there is an initial vocant followed by the same pharyngeal friction sound as before, though on a shorter time scale. This is repeated a second later and a second after that, despite the mother's utterance at M.3 (perhaps because the necessary neuro-vocal organization had already taken place) the child produces his second vocant-closant-vocant (VCV) combination, with slight alteration of the initial vocant and a more pronounced second pulse, "ar ger". This vocal behaviour is almost certainly a foreshadowing of syllabic structure. A further point of interest is that though this child (and the others) has since soon after birth often been producing sounds with an initial "h"-like sound preceding the vocant (*i.e.* a CV pattern), the first sounds which have a more specifically speech-like quality to them show a VCV pattern, which is not a prominent feature of adult speech.

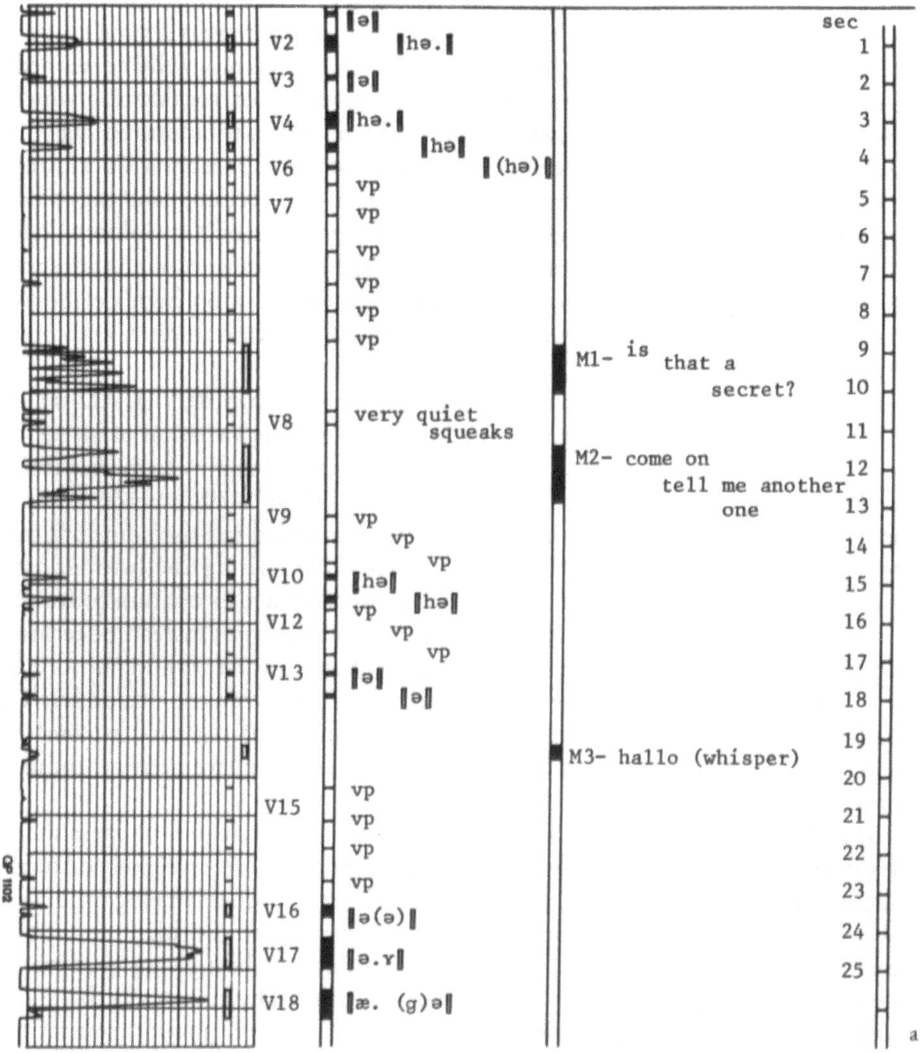

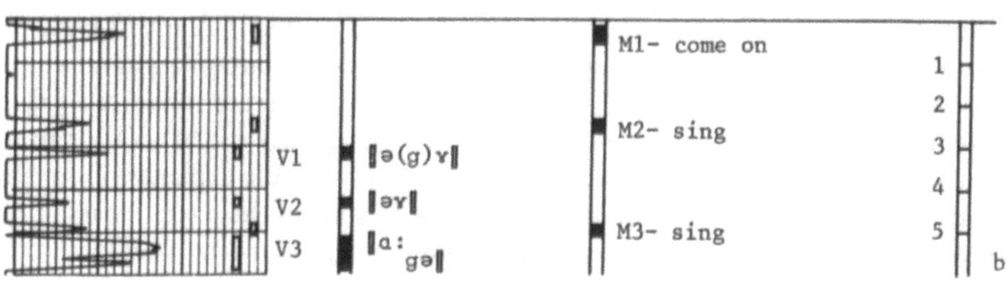

Fig. 4.10 a and b

8. Rosi 3.5 M

The vocal patterning which was becoming apparent in the previous time section and was just detectable in Rosi at 26 days in its earliest form is now fully developed. She has finished a feed and is engaged in a long sequence of vocalization which holds her parents' attention and which they make no effort to interrupt. Fig. 4.11 shows the considerable vocal activity a child can produce in 30 seconds. Vocal panting occurs and in fact was the immediate precursor of this section, ushering in her long monologue: the tape-recorded material reveals evidence of it in children up to 15 months. There is however a notable scarcity of the brief vocant sounds noted in all the previous sections. This behaviour has been replaced by more highly elaborated vocalizations which are of long duration, marked variation in pitch and loudness, and with an increased range of vocant sounds.

The mean duration of the seven sounds V.2, V.3, V.4, V.5, V.10, V.11, V.12 is 1.28 sec, the longest sound V.10 being sustained for 2.27 sec. The variation of intensity can be clearly seen in the figure and introduces a segmented quality to the vocalizations in which it occurs, *e.g.* V.3, V.4, V.10. The variation in pitch is perceptually a salient feature; V.11 and V.12 for instance show well marked fall-rise contours, the latter vocalization starting at 700 Hz, falling to 400 Hz and rising finally to 520 Hz. It is inappropriate to call such tonal variations in an utterance intonation contours, because of the linguistic significance of the term, and they will instead be termed pitch contours. It is clear that the child is playing in an exploratory and purposeful way with the sounds she is making and one can only emphasize a conclusion arrived at earlier, that these vocalizations may in no way simply be regarded as comfort sounds. The child is engaged in a much more serious cognitive activity, though showing every sign of enjoying it at the same time.

In addition to exploring variation, and so control, of pitch and loudness she is also exploring the range of vocant sounds she can produce. It is extremely difficult to identify the different vocants, partly because they are probably being produced in ways which differ from an adult speaker. One cannot be confident about the accuracy of the transcription, which should be regarded as at best giving an approximate indication of the sound values of the vocants uttered by children at this stage of vocal development. It is possible to be rather more confident about the variation in value of these sounds, at least within the temporal limits of duration of normally spoken vowels. A narrower, more precise transcription would probably add nothing further to our understanding. The VCV pattern already noted is clearly in evidence, as in V.3 and V.4. The closant sound is a long-continued palato-pharyngeal voiced fricative ⟦ɣ::⟧ or throaty "ghhh" whilst in V.2 there is also an unvoiced ⟦x⟧ or "(k)hhh". There may be a succession of vocants alone, giving rise to a VVV pattern such as "ah-eh-er" in V.5 or "ah-wer-ah" in V.11. The probable explanation for this vocal behaviour is that the child is learning how to control the overall mass of the tongue for vocal as opposed to feeding purposes, keeping it relatively low in the floor of the mouth with the mouth moderately open, and with some ability to move the mass of the tongue a little forward, or back towards the soft palate and posterior pharyngeal wall. It is interesting that the child explores variation in vocants well before closants. Whether this is because the adult's vowels are percep-

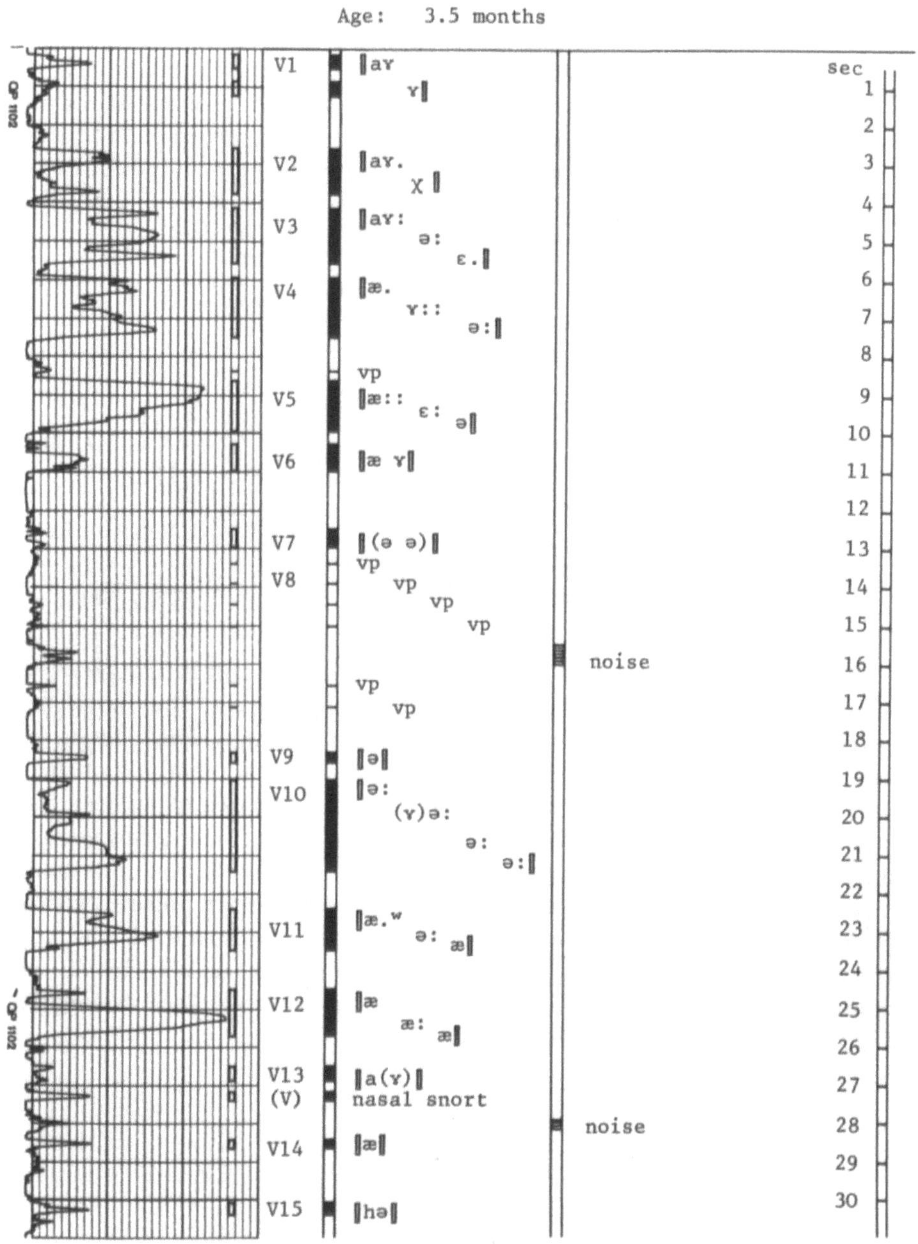

Fig. 4.11

tually salient or because neuromotor organization is more effective for control of the musculature of the body of the tongue is entirely a matter for conjecture at this point in time. In any case the one might imply or explain the other.

9. Helen; English, girl 4.5 M

The vocal behaviour demonstrated in the previous section is now brought to a high state of perfection. To put it in context, Fig. 4.12 represents 15 seconds out of a prolonged sequence in which the child's vocal behaviour is being carried on as an activity in its own right, with a momentum which defies her mother to interrupt even if she wanted to. During this period of vocalization which lasted for 102 sec, there were 39 vocalizations; the data are best presented in tabular form.

Table 4.2. *Summary of vocalization data in a child aged 4.5 M*

Vocalizations:	Duration of vocal activity	102 sec
	Number of vocalizations	39
	Total duration of vocalizations	51.5 sec
	Mean duration of each vocalization	1.32 sec; SD 0.85 sec
	Mean occurrence rate of a vocalization	every 2.6 sec
	Rate of vocalizations per minute	23
Pulses:	Total number of sound pulses	117
	Mean number of pulses per vocalization	3
	Rate of pulse production (whilst vocalizing)	2.3 per sec

The section itself shows a particularly exuberant series of vocalizations taken from the whole sequence. The changes in intensity are readily apparent, and the extent of her exploration of vocant sounds is shown by the transcription. The sequence as a whole has a rather tense, throaty quality probably revealing something of the intense effort the child was putting into her vocal activity. An attempt has been made to indicate this quality for those vocants where it is particularly marked by using the phonetic symbol for pharyngeal friction, /ɤ/ as a subscript. V.6 shows this quality and also shows the remarkable length (3.23 sec) and intricate pulsing, with six individual pulses apparent to the listener, which a child is capable of at this age. Variation in pitch is prominent, and certain patterns recur, *e.g.* V.3. For V.3 with a duration of 1.8 sec the pitch values at approximately every 0.3 sec starting with 210 Hz are 230—440—510—490—520—350 Hz.

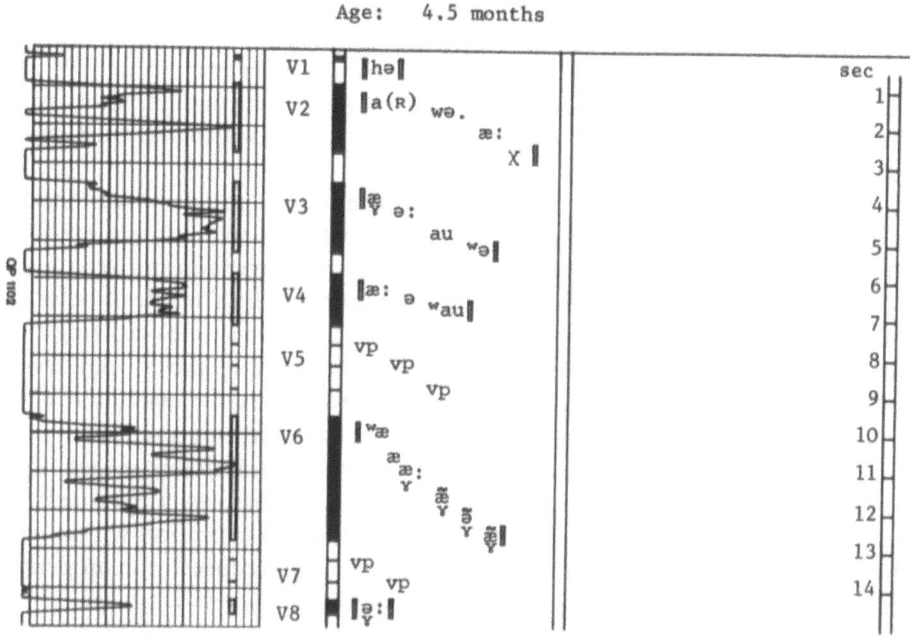

Fig. 4.12

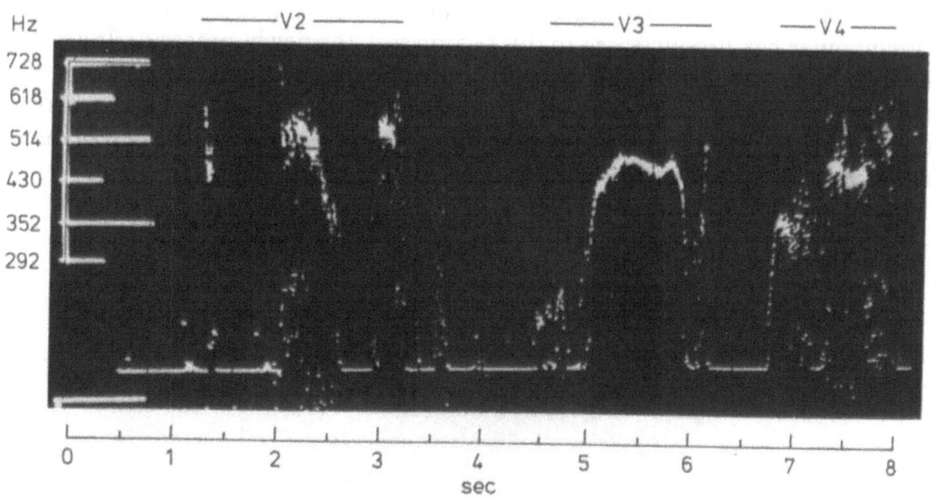

Fig. 4.13. Vocal pitch. Age 4.5 M; showing range of pitch change in a single utterance, and differing pitch contours in successive utterances

10. Matt; Father, Chagga from Northern Tanzania, boy Mother, Muganda from Central Uganda 5.5 M

This boy was born in Kampala, and as his father worked there in the University, the child was exposed mostly to Luganda, a Bantu language, which was the first language of his two older sisters.

Fig. 4.14 ushers in a new stage of development, though one which depends very clearly on the level of control of the vocal apparatus previously achieved. The child's exuberant use of loudness and pitch change no longer appears to be an end in itself, but these features are modulated much more finely. The rate of pulse production during vocal activity rises in consequence, in this example occurring at the rate of 167 per min though this is only a moderate increase over the rate of 138 vocal pulses per minute in Section 9. These features contribute to the qualitative difference in the pattern of vocalization now produced, but the major component of the difference is the greatly increased range and use of vocant and closant sounds. It will be convenient from now on to refer to these sounds collectively as phonants, the term being used for the segmental sounds of a child's vocalization which, when they have passed through the intermediate stage preceding speech can properly be called phonemes, concomitant with the appearance of spoken language.

The child is using a repertoire of 6 vocants, no differentiation here being made between shorter and longer vocants of the same quality. The vocant identified most frequently is [[æ]], which occurred 23 times in the section, followed by [[u]], a vocant which had not previously been heard, and [[ə]]. The identification of these vocant sounds especially will reflect one's own linguistically generated perceptual bias. The closant range has also increased in this section to 4, the newly appearing [[b]] being used on 16 occasions, with [[g]] somewhat surprisingly trailing the field since it was the first closant after [[h]] to be used. There is an underlying palato-pharyngeal frictional quality [[ɣ]] to a number of vocalizations. The numerical data are best presented once again in tabular form.

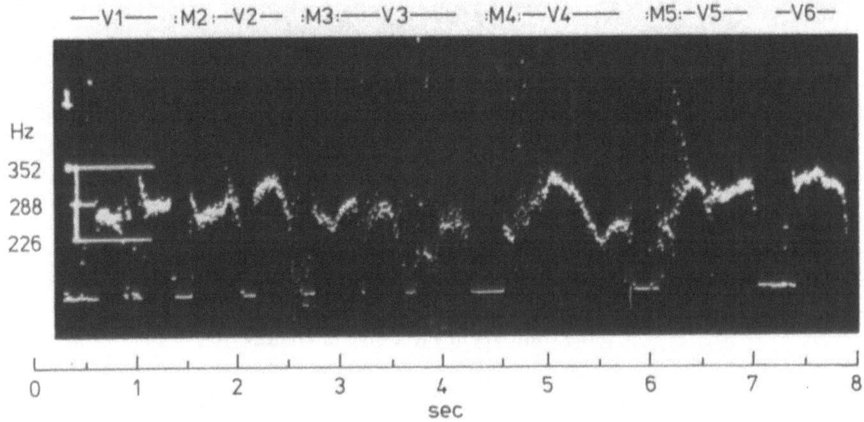

Fig. 4.15. Vocal pitch. Age 5.5 M; in close vocal interaction with mother, sharing her pitch range and showing precise control of pitch contours

Age: 5.5 months

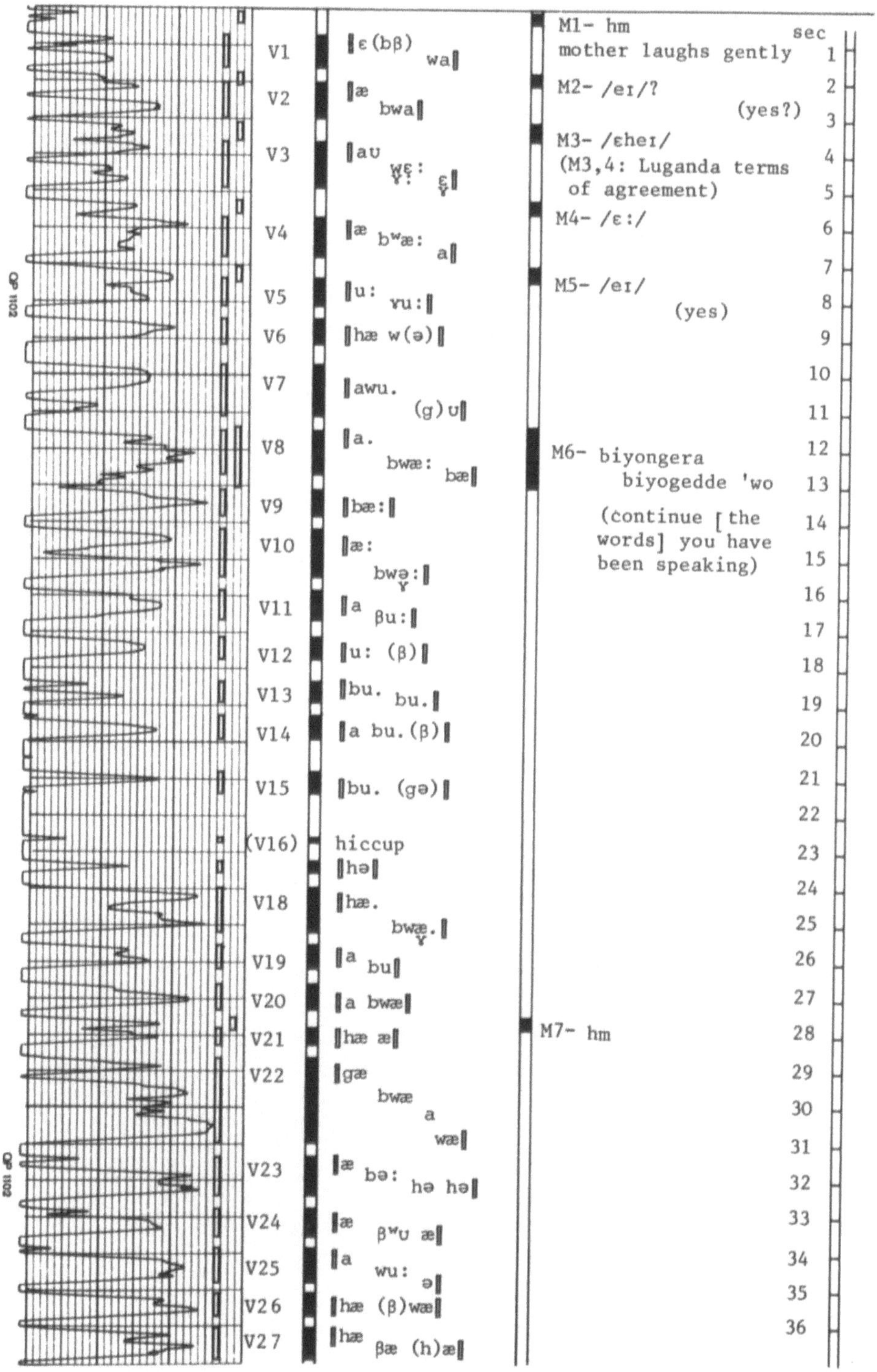

Fig. 4.14

It will be seen from Table 4.3 that the child's rate of pulse and phonant production during his vocalizing activity is, at 5.5 M, surprisingly close to that which an adult speaker shows for syllable and phoneme production.

An additional point of interest is that this child is vocalizing in a way which is now subtly different from the English speaking children, and is using stress, pitch contours and phonant patterns which begin to reflect his mother tongue.

Table 4.3. *Summary of vocalization data in a child aged 5.5 M*

	Duration of section	37 sec
Vocalization:	Number of child vocalizations	26
	Duration of vocalizations	19.8 sec
	Mean duration of a vocalization	0.76 sec; SD 0.41 sec
Pulses:	Total number of vocal pulses	55
	Mean number of pulses per vocalization	2.1
	Duration of a pulse	0.36 sec
	Rate of pulse production	2.8 per sec (168 per m)
Phonants:	Total number of phonants	109
	Range: Vocants 6; Closants 4; Intermediants, [[w]] 1	
	Mean number of phonants per pulse	2.0
	Mean duration of a phonant	0.18 sec
	Rate of phonant production whilst vocalizing	5.6 per sec

11. Peter 6.0 M

The role of a child's siblings and their value in helping the development of communication skills and the acquisition of language have not received the consideration they deserve. Fig. 4.16 is included to give an indication of the extent of their involvement. The child had been got ready for bed and left with his elder sister, Sarah, aged 5 years 7 months; there had been a good deal of vocal interaction between the two, the tail end of which is seen in his sister's utterances S. 1–3. The child's excitement begins to subside concomitant with their mother appearing to put him to bed. At that point his sister invents another game, and holding his feet claps them together. The rhythmical clapping and speaking give the child further enjoyment and he responds with simple pleasurable vocalizations. His sister increases the complexity of her timing, coordinating very precisely her vocalizing and clapping movements; it would be interesting to know whether the rhythmical patterning was modulated primarily by her speech rhythms or by the physical activity. As no doubt she had intended, the result is the greatly increased enjoyment of the child as may be seen in his increased vocalization accompanying this development and his final chuckle.

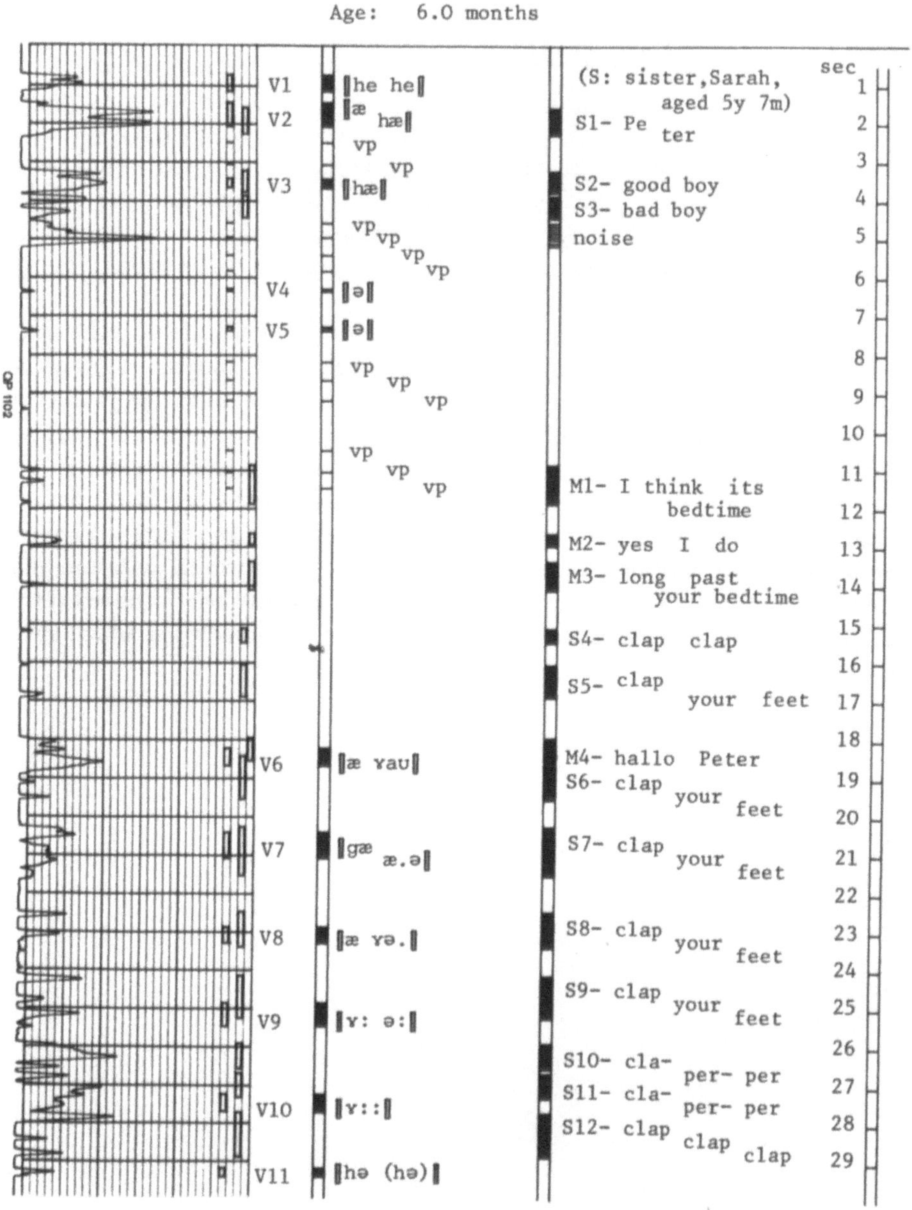
Age: 6.0 months
V1
‖he he‖
V2
‖æ hæ‖
vp
vp
V3
‖hæ‖
vp vp vp vp
V4
‖ə‖
V5
‖ə‖
vp vp vp
vp vp vp
V6
‖æ ɣaʊ‖
V7
‖gæ æ.ə‖
V8
‖æ ɣə.‖
V9
‖ɣ: ə:‖
V10
‖ɣ::‖
V11
‖hə (hə)‖
(S: sister,Sarah, aged 5y 7m)
S1- Pe ter
S2- good boy
S3- bad boy
noise
M1- I think its bedtime
M2- yes I do
M3- long past your bedtime
S4- clap clap
S5- clap your feet
M4- hallo Peter
S6- clap your feet
S7- clap your feet
S8- clap your feet
S9- clap your feet
S10- cla- per- per
S11- cla- per- per
S12- clap clap clap
sec
1
2
3
4
5
6
7
8
9
10
11
12
13
14
15
16
17
18
19
20
21
22
23
24
25
26
27
28
29
QP 1102

Fig. 4.16

12. Matt 7.6 M

There is no new vocal behaviour in Fig. 4.17; if anything it is suggestive of vocal activity earlier than that of the previous (5.5 M) section for the tempo of its production. It is however more restrained and the pitch contours show much less variation, V.7 for instance being held at 300 Hz for the greater part of its length with a rise of 350 Hz at the beginning of the final pulse starting with "h" and falling to 270 Hz. There is a suggestion of two new vocants [[o]] and [[i]], but there is an almost complete absence of closants which no doubt in part accounts for its rather younger quality.

There are two features of special interest relating to his voice and the interaction. Throughout the whole duration of the recording he is adopting a low growling voice, and an attempt has been made to indicate this effect by the [[R]] subscript, representing a very light, sustained palato-pharyngeal roughening or trill. The child and his mother consider it highly amusing, and she is reduced several times to giggles prior to the section reproduced in the figure. In the section her behaviour has altered a little, and she is enticing him on. This is shown by her utterance at M.1 after he had quietened down somewhat, an utterance which was an imitation of an earlier sound of his. She imitates him again at M.3, and her brief interjections at M.2, M.4, M.5 are also probably intended to sustain his activity, in which she is highly successful.

Age: 7.6 months

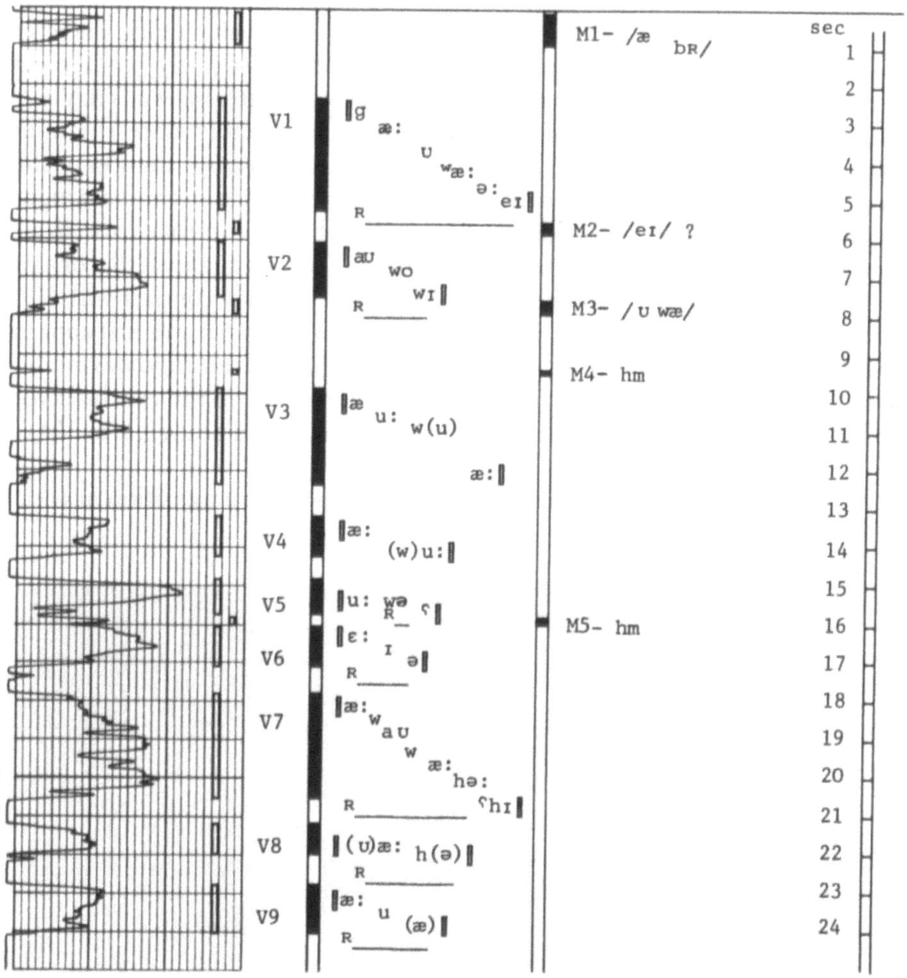

Fig. 4.17

13. Peter 8.5 M

In this section there is an interesting mixture of vocal behaviours. There is for instance the boisterous prolonged vocalization of V.9 strongly reminiscent of Helen at 4.5 M; and some compact, very controlled vocal utterances at V.1, V.6, V.12. The initial vocalization of the section is especially notable since the minutes preceding it were characterized by loud chuckles and shouting cadences of sound, one example of which persisted for 4.2 sec. But interspersed in this very vigorous vocal behaviour there occur occasional brief, quiet, highly controlled vocalizations of which V.1 is an example. Its structure is V-CV-CV and its quality is that of a single spoken word; the same could be said of V.6 and V.12. They contrast with V.3 for instance which is an echo from the days when a VCV utterance was first appearing, the closant being a gentle throaty "ghhh" sound of the type this child was producing at 1.6 M. Other evidence of earlier vocal behaviours is seen in the very brief vocant sound of V.7, and the vocal panting of which there is a good deal, *e.g.* after V.4, V.10, V.11.

It seems possible that we are witnessing in this section a transition in vocal be-

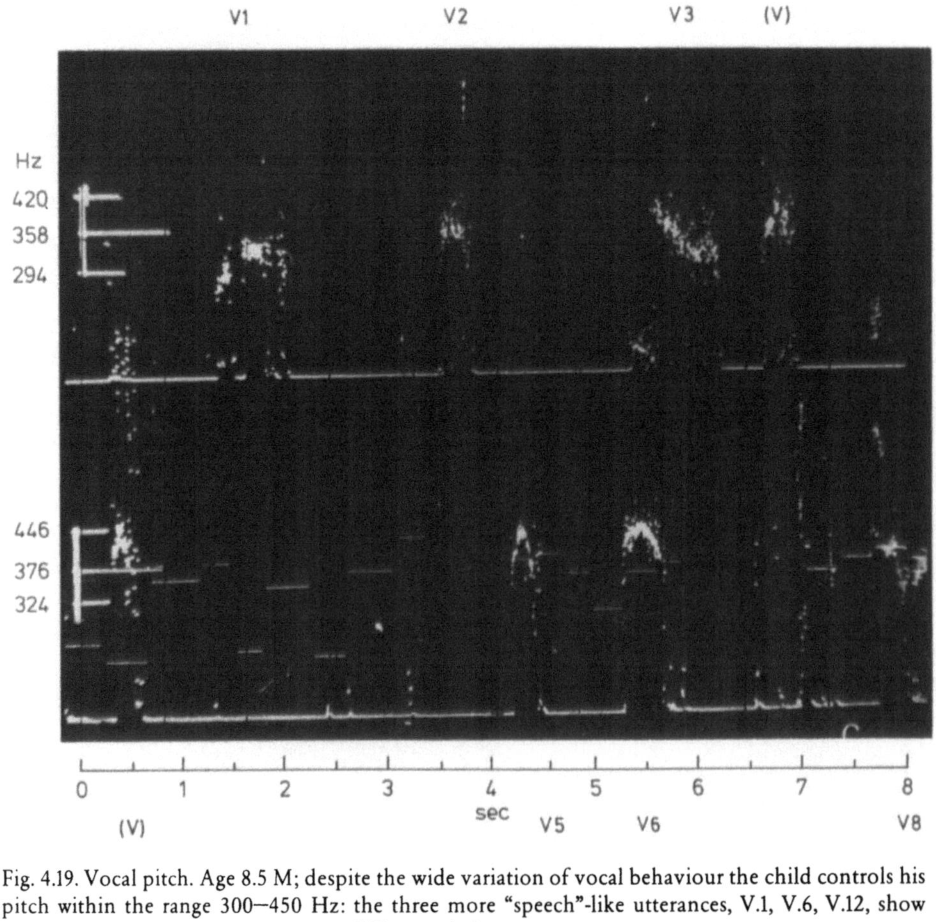

Fig. 4.19. Vocal pitch. Age 8.5 M; despite the wide variation of vocal behaviour the child controls his pitch within the range 300—450 Hz: the three more "speech"-like utterances, V.1, V.6, V.12, show different pitch contours

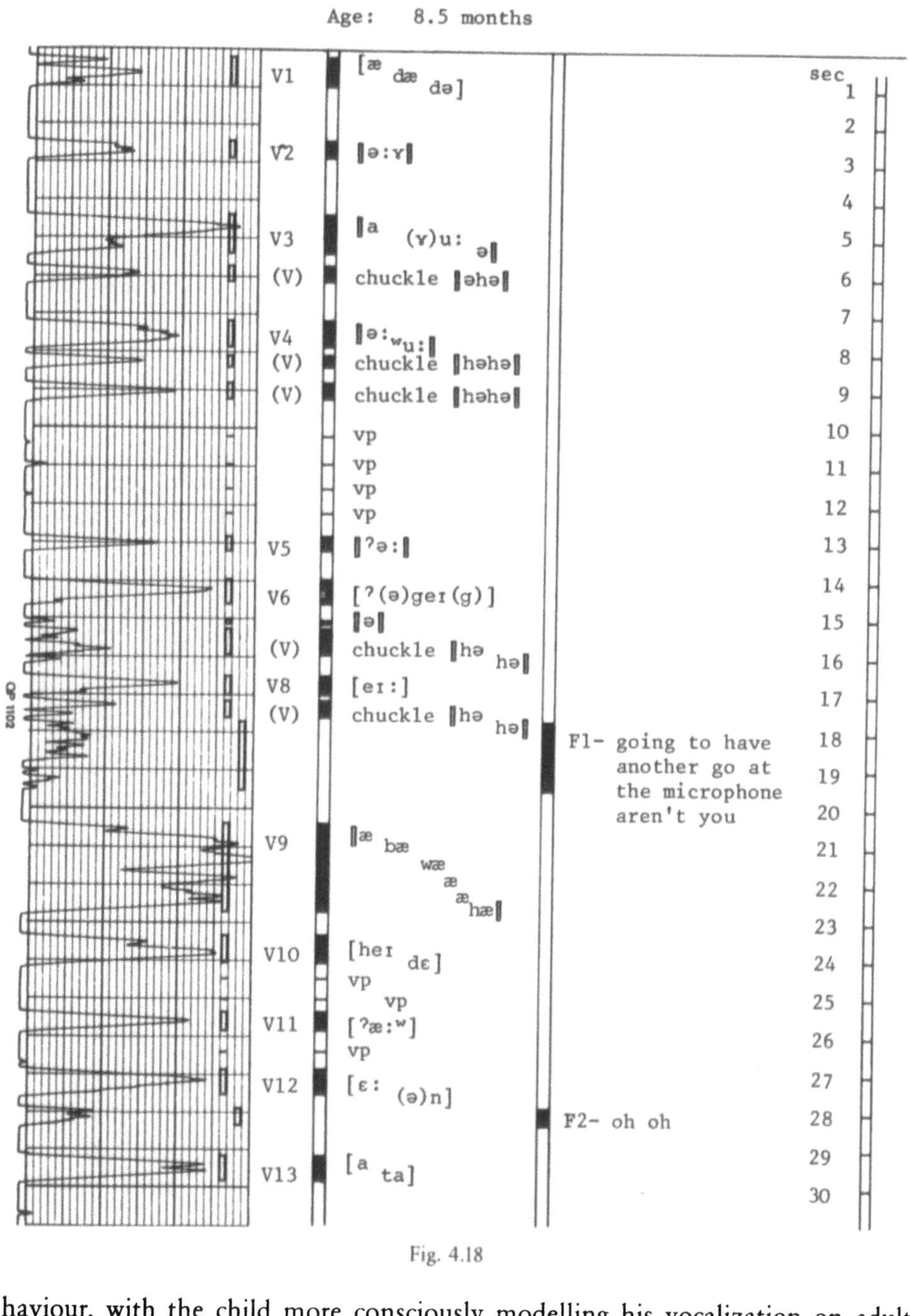

Fig. 4.18

haviour, with the child more consciously modelling his vocalization on adult speech sounds. The closants are better defined and in the figure include "d", "g", "b", "w", "h", "n" and "t". They are becoming more consonant-like and though we may not refer to them as consonants in the absence of linguistic behaviour, we may be justified in labelling them their immediate precursors *i.e.* consonantals. If this is possibly the case for the closants, it is almost certainly true for the vocants, which are becoming more easily identified within the categories of adult speech, and so could be labelled vowelals.

14. Peter 9.4 M

The trend towards shorter individual vocalizations continues. In this section the total duration of vocal activity is 7.8 sec, which with 9 vocalizations gives a mean duration of 0.87 sec. There are 21 pulses of vocal sound, giving a pulse production rate of 2.7 per sec. The impression gained from the recording indicates further increase in control of the vocal apparatus. V.4 illustrates the point. There are two virtually identical pulses of sound, each commencing at 660 Hz and falling in 0.17 sec to 480 Hz. Superimposed on this beautifully modulated carrier wave there is a CV pattern for each of the two pulses, but the child is able to articulate the consonantal [b] to initiate the first pulse, and to change it to [g] for the second. Neuromotor function, sufficient to permit the child to produce a well-defined "b" with the two lips, and change this to "g" with the tongue moving back into contact with soft palate, indicates a remarkable ability to organize and control the sequence of activity, especially whilst retaining such accurate control of respiratory and laryngeal activity.

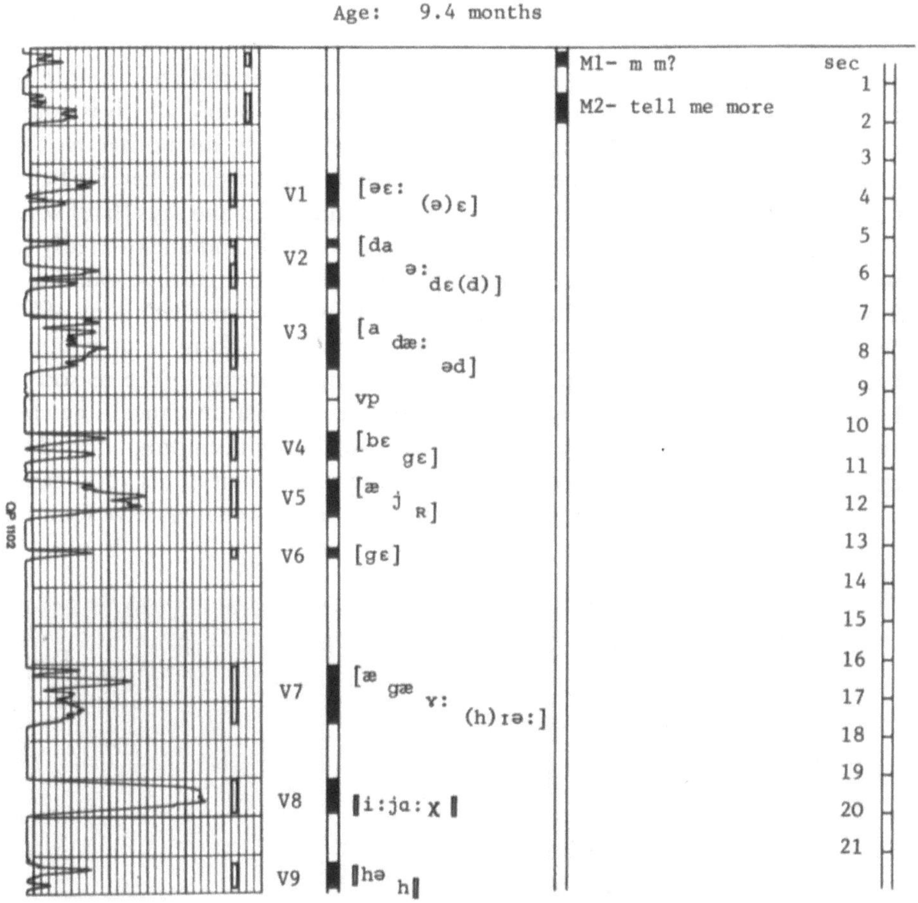
Age: 9.4 months
M1- m m?
M2- tell me more
sec
V1 [əɛ: (ə)ɛ]
V2 [da ə: dɛ(d)]
V3 [a dæ: əd]
vp
V4 [bɛ gɛ]
V5 [æ j ʀ]
V6 [gɛ]
V7 [æ gæ ɣ: (h)ɪə:]
V8 i:ja:χ
V9 hə h
1
2
3
4
5
6
7
8
9
10
11
12
13
14
15
16
17
18
19
20
21

Fig. 4.20

15. Peter 10.1 M

There had already been a long interaction beween mother and child before the start of Fig. 4.21. It starts (M.1) with a long drawnout /"booo"/ which is copied moderately well by the child, which in its turn is copied well by his mother. He then changes the vowelal and says [bɑ:(b)] which is accurately copied by her. He begins to get excited, revealed by the initial ingressive sound of V.3 and says [bəʊ] which his mother copies as "bo-wo". He however has immediately and unexpectedly followed V.3 by V.4, the two only separated by another excited ingressive sound as he quickly draws breath to say [ɑ: bɑ:], which overlaps with his mother's copy of V.3. The mother, possibly disconcerted by his unexpected turn-taking, or uncertain of what is happening, or to damp down the mounting excitement (the reason for which she is as yet unaware) says /m::/ and repeats her last utterance. The child immediately follows her with [a bɑ . . .] as if it had already been programmed but slightly delayed by her utterance, and adds on the second half of his vocalization [. . . wa wa], probably in imitation of her. With another excited ingressive sound he

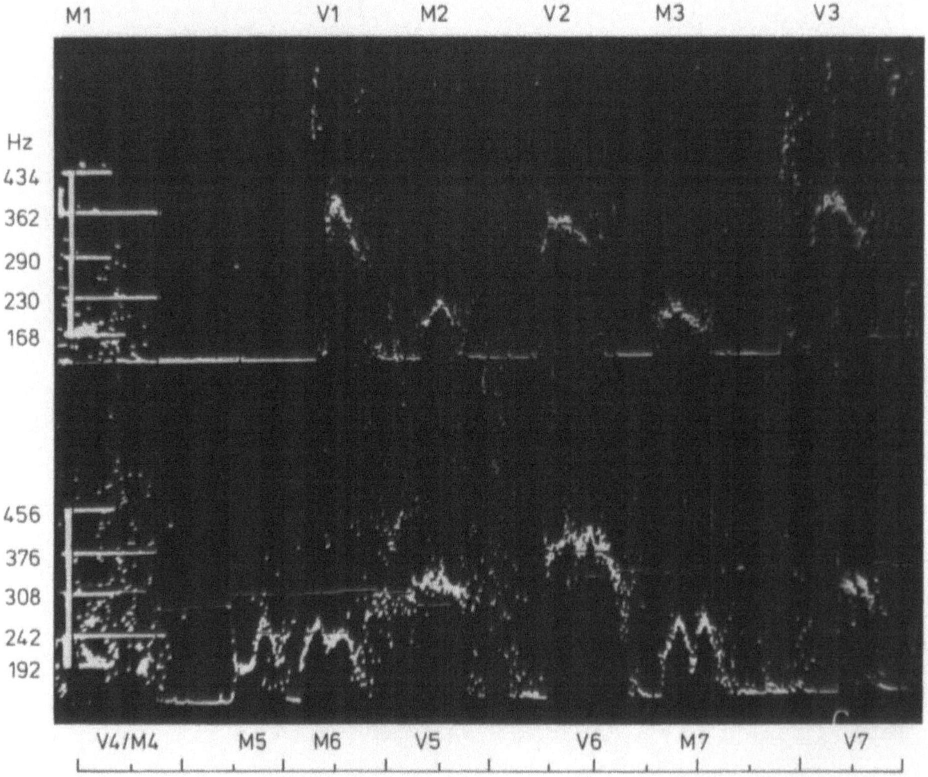

Fig. 4.22. Vocal pitch. Age 10.1 M; the difference in pitch between the child's voice and his mother's is readily apparent, being about $^2/_3$ octave in the upper half of the figure; and there is a remarkable similarity between related pitch contours, *e.g.* V.2 and M.3. Brief high frequency bursts of sound associated with inspiration may be seen at the beginning and end of V.3 and at the end of V.5

Age: 10.1 months

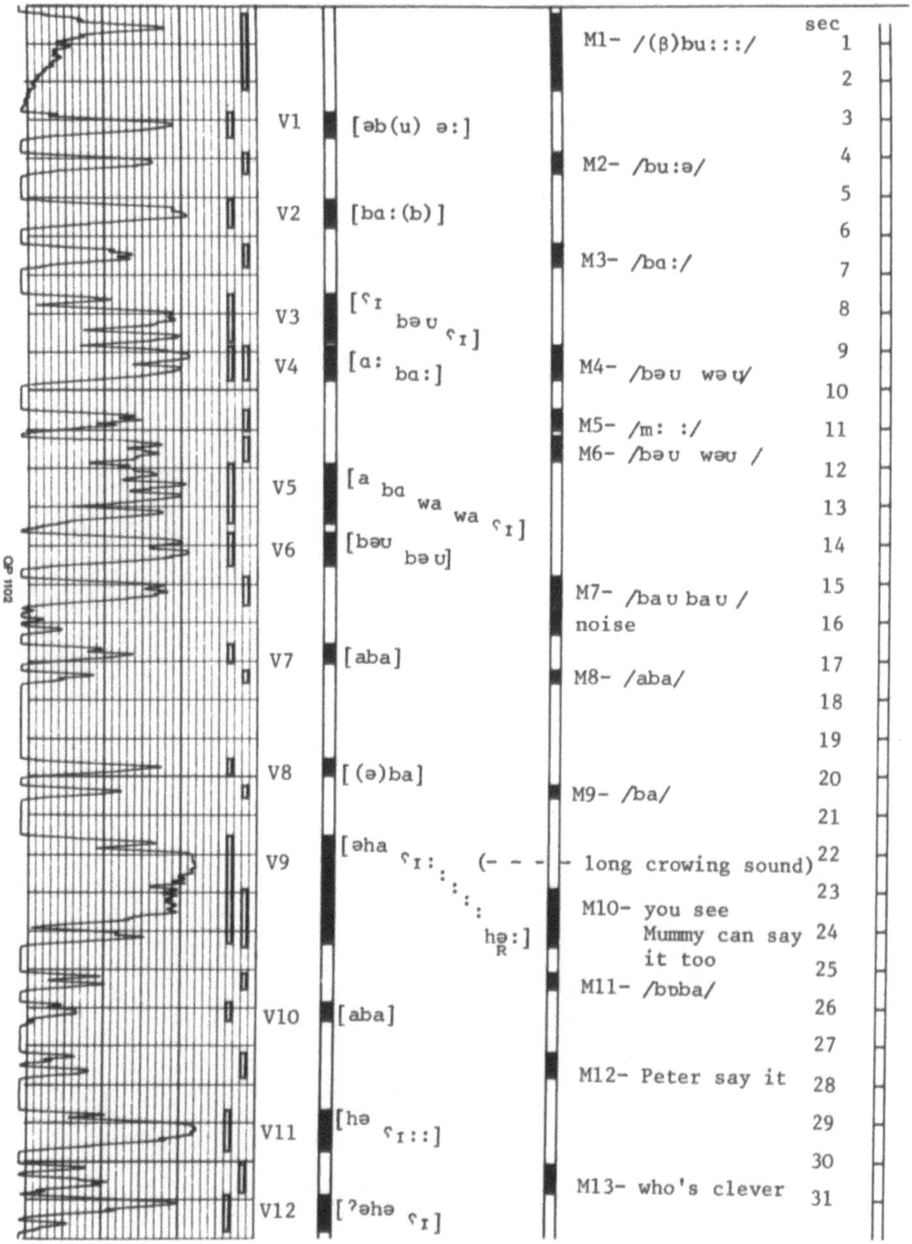

Fig. 4.21

once again jumps her turn and says [bəʊ bəʊ], possibly reverting to V.3, which his mother copies a little inaccurately. The child waits fractionally before his next (usurped) turn at V.7 and says [aba], a pattern which has already been used. This is immediately copied by his mother, who is probably beginning to realize what he is up to, and then the child consciously and deliberately delays his next utterance. This behaviour is revealed by the unusually long silence of 2 sec between her response and his next vocalization V.8, which is [(ə) ba] and which his mother very quickly imitates, showing by her lack of interruption despite the long pause, and her immediate response to him, her acknowledgement of the fact that he has taken over the role of initiator and that she must now follow. He had almost certainly attempted to do this at V.3 and 4 and been thwarted, but tried again without delay at V.5 and 6. Having succeeded not only in taking over her role, but demonstrating unequivocally to her what he has done, his excitement can be contained no longer and he lets out a long triumphant chuckle. After this his mother tries to get the interaction going again, but every time she gives him a model to imitate he simply chuckles, to tease her and remind her how clever he has been, which his mother perceptively acknowledges by saying "Who's clever!".

The details of this brief half-minute of interaction are sufficient to indicate the level of sophistication which is achieved by a child of this age in vocal control, situational awareness, and grasp of the rules of turn-taking. His mastery of these rules and his cognitive development is such that he is able to misuse them, and achieve a high degree of pleasure in the process. With the natural developmental constraints on his motor activity it is doubtful if he could show such an advanced behaviour in any other way. The section carries clear implications for the importance of skillful and sensitive handling of interaction episodes by the child's parents.

At a more mundane level it appears that we were justified in deciding in the previous section that the child had moved into a more advanced stage of vocal development, and that he probably was producing truly vowel-like and consonant-like sounds. The child's imitation of his mother's speech sounds and the subsequent play centred around them suggest that these copies were perceptually acceptable to her and lying within the field of normal speech sounds.

16. Matt 11.1 M

The child's control of the vocal apparatus and of the vocal carrier wave is at the high level of fine-tuning seen already in the section for 9.4 M. But he is now putting his vocalization ability to a more advanced, speech-like use. Whilst the recordist (R) is talking to Prisca (P), a young female relative of the child's mother, the child is constantly interjecting short utterances. They are predominantly vowelals, and are unmistakably of the same nature as a Luganda speaker would use if he or she were listening to a conversation, and expressing interest and affirmation with a non-verbal "eeh", typical of the language. It is as if he is participating in the conversation, signifying his presence and interest. As the adults become aware of this their conversation dies away and his single-pulsed utterances become more complex, but still delicate and restrained, with a simple, repetitive babble pattern appearing briefly at V.13. This is picked up by the recordist 4 seconds later (R.5) but the child does not repeat it, replying instead with a highly characteristic Luganda response in V.17 to his question "Ogamba otya?" *i.e.* "How (what) are you saying?".

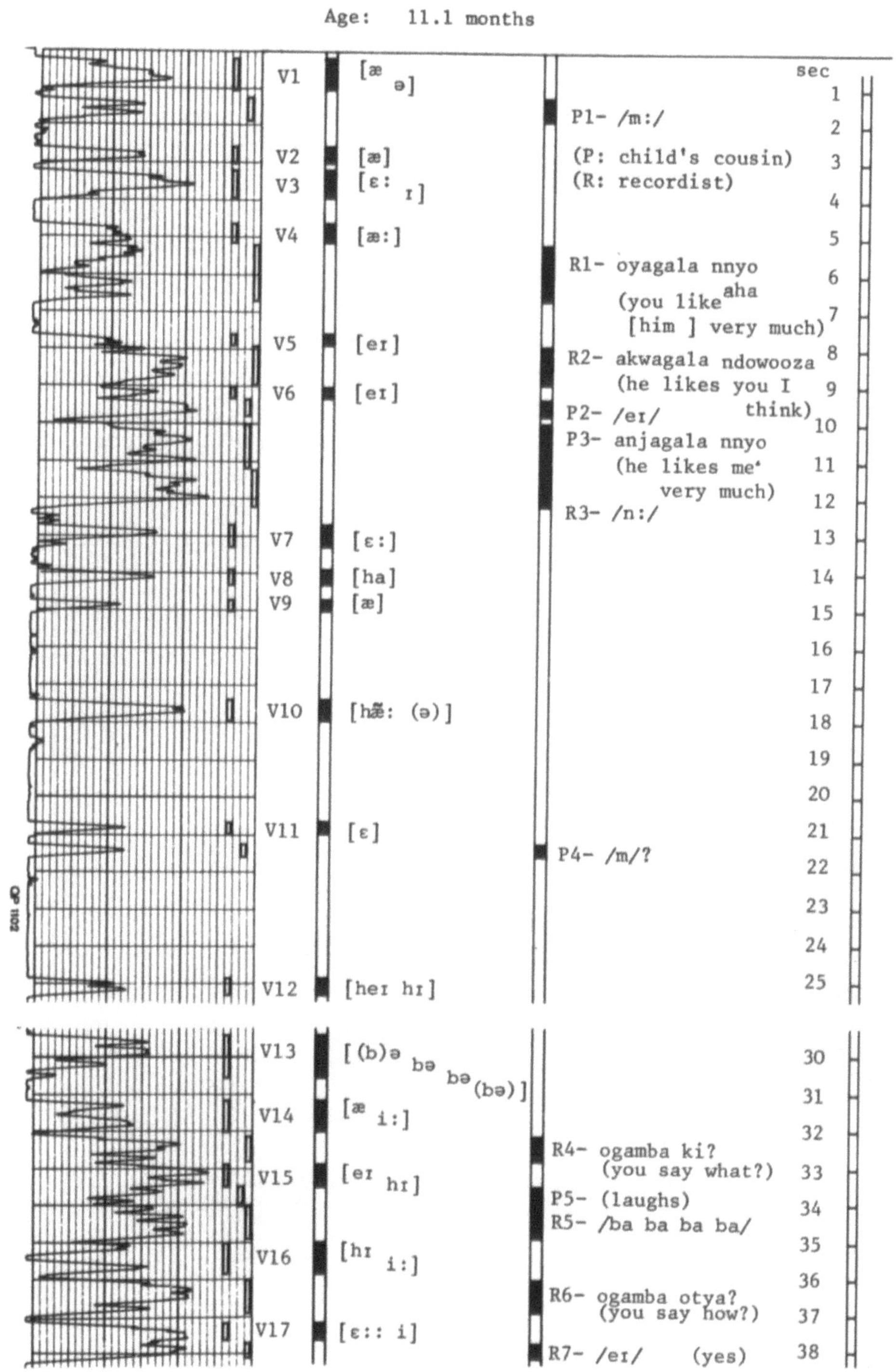
Age: 11.1 months
sec
V1 [æ ə]
P1- /m:/
V2 [æ]
(P: child's cousin)
V3 [ɛ: ɪ]
(R: recordist)
V4 [æ:]
R1- oyagala nnyo
(you like aha [him] very much)
V5 [eɪ]
R2- akwagala ndowooza
(he likes you I think)
V6 [eɪ]
P2- /eɪ/
P3- anjagala nnyo
(he likes me very much)
R3- /n:/
V7 [ɛ:]
V8 [ha]
V9 [æ]
V10 [hæ̃: (ə)]
V11 [ɛ]
P4- /m/?
V12 [heɪ hɪ]
V13 [(b)ə bə bə (bə)]
V14 [æ i:]
R4- ogamba ki?
(you say what?)
V15 [eɪ hɪ]
P5- (laughs)
R5- /ba ba ba ba/
V16 [hɪ i:]
R6- ogamba otya?
(you say how?)
V17 [ɛ:: i]
R7- /eɪ/ (yes)
1
2
3
4
5
6
7
8
9
10
11
12
13
14
15
16
17
18
19
20
21
22
23
24
25
30
31
32
33
34
35
36
37
38

Fig. 4.23

17. Peter 12.4 M

From now on the examples will be taken from this child to maintain continuity and so that the orderly emergence of one ordinary child's speech and early language can be examined. All the previous examples and these should be considered as illustrative of the normal pattern of vocal and speech development, giving the details of how individual children used their voices at specified ages. The stage has not yet been reached when a definitive statement can be made on vocal development and language acquisition, with the incorporation of statistical data relevant to the numerous factors, some known, some as yet unidentified, which contribute to the variation in performance between one child and another.

Fig. 4.24 shows an important development in the use of the voice. It is characterized by very emphatic pulses of vowelal sound, preceded at V.1 by a strange, harsh unvoiced sound, represented [[hx]], which gives the impression that the child had mistimed, and had initiated sharp expiratory airflow before he had

Age: 12.4 months (a)

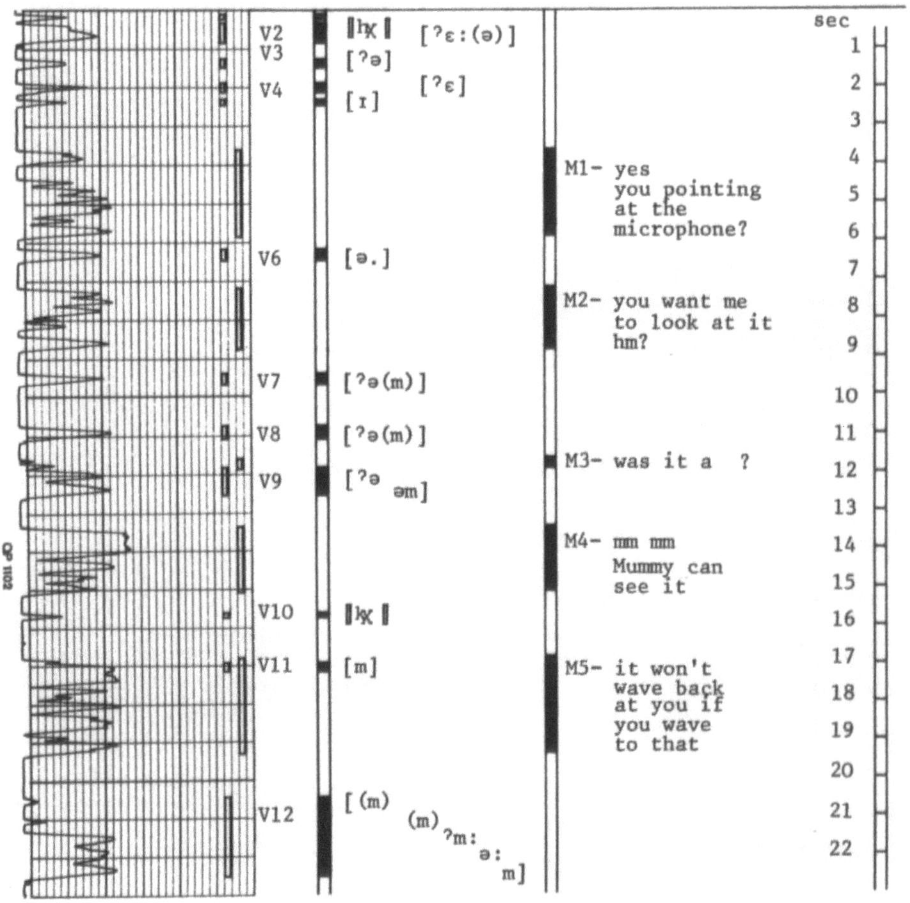

Fig. 4.24 a

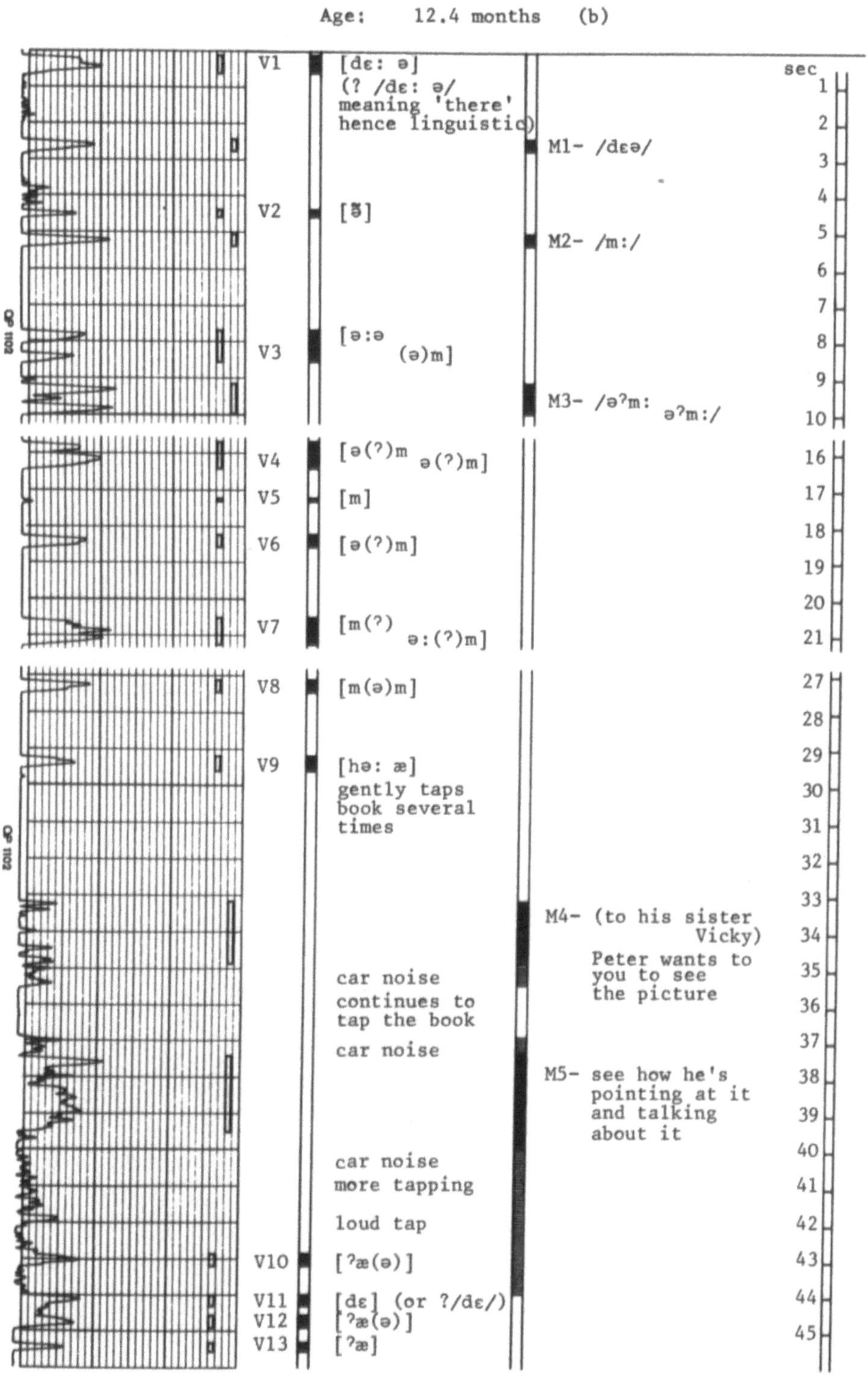
Age: 12.4 months (b)
V1 [dɛ: ə]
(? /dɛ: ə/
meaning 'there'
hence linguistic)
M1- /dɛə/
V2 [ə̃]
M2- /m:/
V3 [ə:ə (ə)m]
M3- /əʔm: əʔm:/
V4 [ə(ʔ)m ə(ʔ)m]
V5 [m]
V6 [ə(ʔ)m]
V7 [m(ʔ) ə:(ʔ)m]
V8 [m(ə)m]
V9 [hə: æ]
gently taps
book several
times
M4- (to his sister
Vicky)
Peter wants to
you to see
the picture
car noise
continues to
tap the book
car noise
M5- see how he's
pointing at it
and talking
about it
car noise
more tapping
loud tap
V10 [ʔæ(ə)]
V11 [dɛ] (or ?/dɛ/)
V12 [ʔæ(ə)]
V13 [ʔæ]
sec
1
2
3
4
5
6
7
8
9
10
16
17
18
19
20
21
27
28
29
30
31
32
33
34
35
36
37
38
39
40
41
42
43
44
45

Fig. 4.24 b

adducted the vocal folds. That this might be the explanation is suggested by the sharp plosive quality of the subsequent vocalizations, V.2–4, a quality which is indicated by the use of the initial glottal stop for each of them, *e.g.* [ʔə]. They have a highly emphatic sound to them as if they are the vocal equivalent of pointing with the finger, and this is confirmed by the mother's comment-question (M.1) about pointing at the microphone, to which he gives an affirmative vocalization. The vocal gesturing behaviour is repeated in V.7–9. This changes after her comment about the microphone not waving back (M.5) and he gives an affirmative, drawn-out and knowing "mm", as if he had understood perfectly, but in fact responding to the declarative intonation contour of her utterance.

(b) occurred two minutes later in the same session, whilst he was looking at a picture in a book. At M.5 his mother says "See how he's pointing at it and talking about it". He taps the book several times with his finger, then gives it an extra firm tap and accompanies this with a highly emphatic plosive vowelal sound once again, to be followed by [dɛ]. This is a sound which has recently appeared and from its sound and the occasions on which he uses it is suggestive of "there", as at the beginning of this section, V.1.

The use to which the child is putting his voice in this recording gives the impression that it is bordering on the linguistic. He is uttering sounds which are almost becoming conventionalized or stereotyped in order to convey information to his mother, and the reciprocity of vocal and manual gesturing is revealing. Fig. 4.24 b shows him taking this a little further as he follows the vocal and hand gestures with a word-like utterance, which could well be a delayed imitation of the numerous occasions he has heard his mother and others use "there" in similar situations. The final, and perhaps most important point, is that he is not responsive as in the previous section, but is very much the initiator in these speech-like acts.

18. Peter 14.0 M

Fig. 4.25 shows the emergence of highly organized vocal behaviour at the segmental level, that is of the individual speech-like vowelals and consonantals which we might refer to collectively as phonals. There is an increase in the range of phonals; the child is able to use different groupings of phonals in consecutive vocalizations; his patterning of the pulses of vocal carrier wave sound, and the stress these are given can seemingly be changed at will; and the arrangement of phonals shows considerable voluntary variation. All this may be seen in the first six vocalizations of the figure.

His range of phonals is seen to be, for the vowelals—[æ], [e], [eɪ] (a diphthong), [ɪ], [a], [ɔ], [ə], [ʌ]; for the consonantals—[v], [d], [t], [g]; and for the intermedials (if we may use this term to refer to the pre-speech equivalents of the consonants which show no closure or marked constriction of the vocal tract, and which are classed variously as nasals, laterals, semi-vowels, and continuants) there are [m], [l] and [j].

Each of the vocalizations V.1, 2, 4, and 5 is in effect a different utterance because of the range of phonals which each contains, none of them being similar in this respect. The first three of these vocalizations contain 3 pulses, though the temporal arrangement of these within each vocalization is different, and V.5 shows no less than 11 and possibly 12 pulses. The stress, which is essentially a perceptual phenomenon and is not simply a function of intensity (Fry, 1958), also shows a varying pattern. If we label a weak or unstressed pulse "0", a moderate stress "1", and a strong stress "2", the pulse stress (S) is S (1 2 0) for V.1; for V.2, S (1 1 1); for V.4, S (0 0 1); and V.5 shows no specially stressed pulse, as for V.2.

The sequential arrangement of segmental sounds has been surprisingly neglected. It is at least as important a feature of developing speech as the order of emergence of individual sounds, since no single phonant or phonal (or phoneme either for that matter) can have more than an infinitesimal significance when it occurs as an isolated vocal event. It is the rule-bound ordering of a mere 44 phonemes (for English) which permits the generation of hundreds of thousands of words, the total being limitless. To return to the limitations of this child's vocalizations, it can be seen that definite patterns of sequence are present, and that it is not purely random vocal activity as has been asserted. Sequences of segmental sounds are probably best analyzed by looking at each successive pair and determining the combinations of sounds which occur, and the number of times such pairings take place. This may be done using a transition matrix, in which the first sound of the pair is identified across the rows and the second down the colmns. The use of an example will make the procedure clear, and it was devised specifically to see if identifiable patterns of sound production occur in so-called jargon, such as V.5.

[ə. d ʌ g l d (ə) g l a d l a d l a d l a d l ə d l (ə)] ... V.5

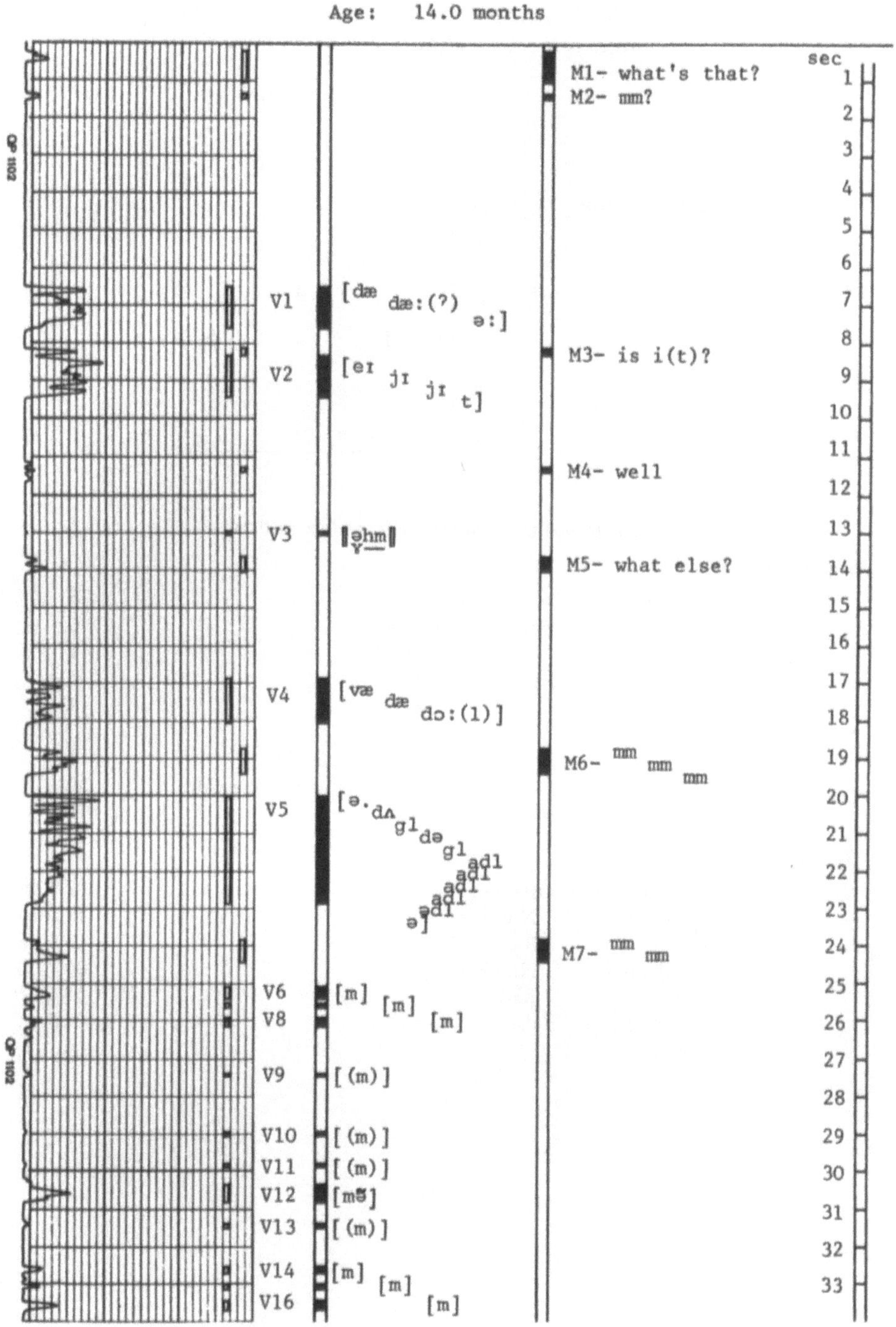

Age: 14.0 months
sec
V1 [dæ dæ:(?) ə:]
V2 [eɪ jɪ jɪ t]
V3
V4 [væ dæ dɔ:(1)]
V5 [ə·dʌ gl də gl adl adl adl adl ə]
V6 [m] [m] [m]
V8
V9 [(m)]
V10 [(m)]
V11 [(m)]
V12
V13 [(m)]
V14 [m] [m] [m]
V16
M1- what's that?
M2- mm?
M3- is i(t)?
M4- well
M5- what else?
M6- mm mm mm
M7- mm mm
1
2
3
4
5
6
7
8
9
10
11
12
13
14
15
16
17
18
19
20
21
22
23
24
25
26
27
28
29
30
31
32
33

Fig. 4.25

Table 4.4 a. *Transition matrix for jargon string of vocalization V.5 (from Fig. 4.25) showing occurrence rate of phonal pairs. For details see text*

First phonal \ Second phonal	ə	ʌ	a	d	g	l
ə				2	1	
ʌ					1	
a				4		
d	1	1				5
g						2
l	2		4	1		

Table 4.4 b. *Analysis of transition matrix*

1. Segmental features			
	Total number of phonals		25
	Number of phonal types	(single)	6
		(paired)	11
	Occurrence rate of pairs:	dl	5
		ad, la	4
		əd, gl, lə	2
		əg, ʌg, də, dʌ, ld	1
	Number of possible pairs (excluding identical, *e.g.* dd)		30
	Number of pairs not produced		19
2. Temporal features			
	Duration of utterance		2.9 sec
	Pulses:	Number	11 (or 12)
		Rate	3.8 per sec
	Phonals:	Number	25
		Rate	8.6 per sec
	Phonals per pulse		2.3

The individual phonal types are first identified, and these are used to label the rows and columns of the matrix as in Table 4.4 a. To enter the matrix the initial sound of the string [ə] is found in the left hand column, representing the "First phonal" and one travels across this row until the column representing the second phonal [d] is found, from the row of "Second phonal" across the top of the matrix. The occurrence is marked (a convenient method is to number the first pair "1", the second pair "2" and so on), the second phonal now becomes the first of the second pair and the procedure is repeated until all the pairs have been entered. This will be one less than the total number of phonals of the string; in V.5 there are 25 individual sounds, and 24 pairs. The data which result from this procedure and certain associated findings are included in Table 4.4 b. The use of a transition matrix can be extended to consecutive utterances by using a silent sound "ø" to represent the time between the end of one and the beginning of the next utterance.

19. Peter 15.2 M

This time section is characterized by the occurrence of a number of vocal behaviours which convey a strong impression that the child is speaking. In (b) it sounds like a two-element utterance, and in (a) one can only say, though with considerable misgiving, that the utterance sounds as if it contains three elements, with a subject-verb-object structure. These are followed by examples of interaction with his sister, showing a surprising degree of vocal adaptation on her part, and the section finishes with an example of the more typical speech behaviour associated with this age. The subsections are taken in the serial order in which they occurred during the course of a single recording session.

a) Just before Fig. 4.26 starts the child had produced a long, singing vocalization lasting 2.3 sec, rather similar to the behaviour already noted in much younger children. There is then a silence of nearly 3 seconds and the figure shows the sudden appearance of four strong vocal pants. The last occasion this behaviour was in evidence in these sections was in the same child at 8.5 M. Taken together this vocal behaviour is highly suggestive of intense cognitive activity in the stage preparatory to the production of an utterance which is both difficult for the child and important to him. It always seems to be associated with strong communicative intent. Then the utterance appears, basically four-pulsed, but the pattern is somewhat distorted by four "h" sounds (seen in V.1—V.4), perhaps the subsiding vestiges of his intense effort. If these are ignored the stress pattern is S (1 0 2 0). The pitch is very high, the first pulse falling from its initial value of 1010 Hz to 720 Hz, the second with a rise-fall from 870 Hz to 1020 Hz and down again, and a relatively uniform 710 Hz for the final two pulses. V.2, [ai goʔ gæ da] sounds like "I' (ve) go(t) ?carcar or ?dada", but though it is clearly a highly significant utterance to the child the fact (sadly) is that the meaning was totally obscure to the parents at the time.

b) A rather similar pattern of vocal behaviour is seen at V.1 and V.2 in this part of the section. The father asks a question to which the child responds with two small and a third pronounced "h", the latter so strong that it sounds like a snort and has a nasal quality. This is followed by a small fragment of jargon [lɪdlɪ(dl)], so faint as to be almost inaudible. The father repeats his question very gently and out comes the utterance, V.3. This had almost certainly been organized by the time of the father's repeat question, which was probably unnecessary and he no doubt was unaware of what V.1 and V.2 signalled. The four-pulsed utterance /hɪə di: ʤi i:/ is clearly interpreted by the father as referring to a gee-gee or horse, and it is quite impressive that the child manages the affricate /ʤ/, though not for the initial syllable. We are entitled to talk now in linguistic terms, and to use the appropriate nomenclature and transcription—at least for this utterance. Its appearance increases the possibility that the four-pulsed vocalization in 19 (a) was being formulated in the child's mind in a linguistic mode, and this is supported by the evidence of the cognitive effort involved. It seems likely that many such spontaneous speech (or at least speech-like) productions are overlooked by the child's parents, and he may be spurred on to continue his efforts only by his innate propensity to talk reinforced by their general interest and occasional specific recognition. This lack of feedback arising out of non-comprehension may well be a significant factor in the genesis of language

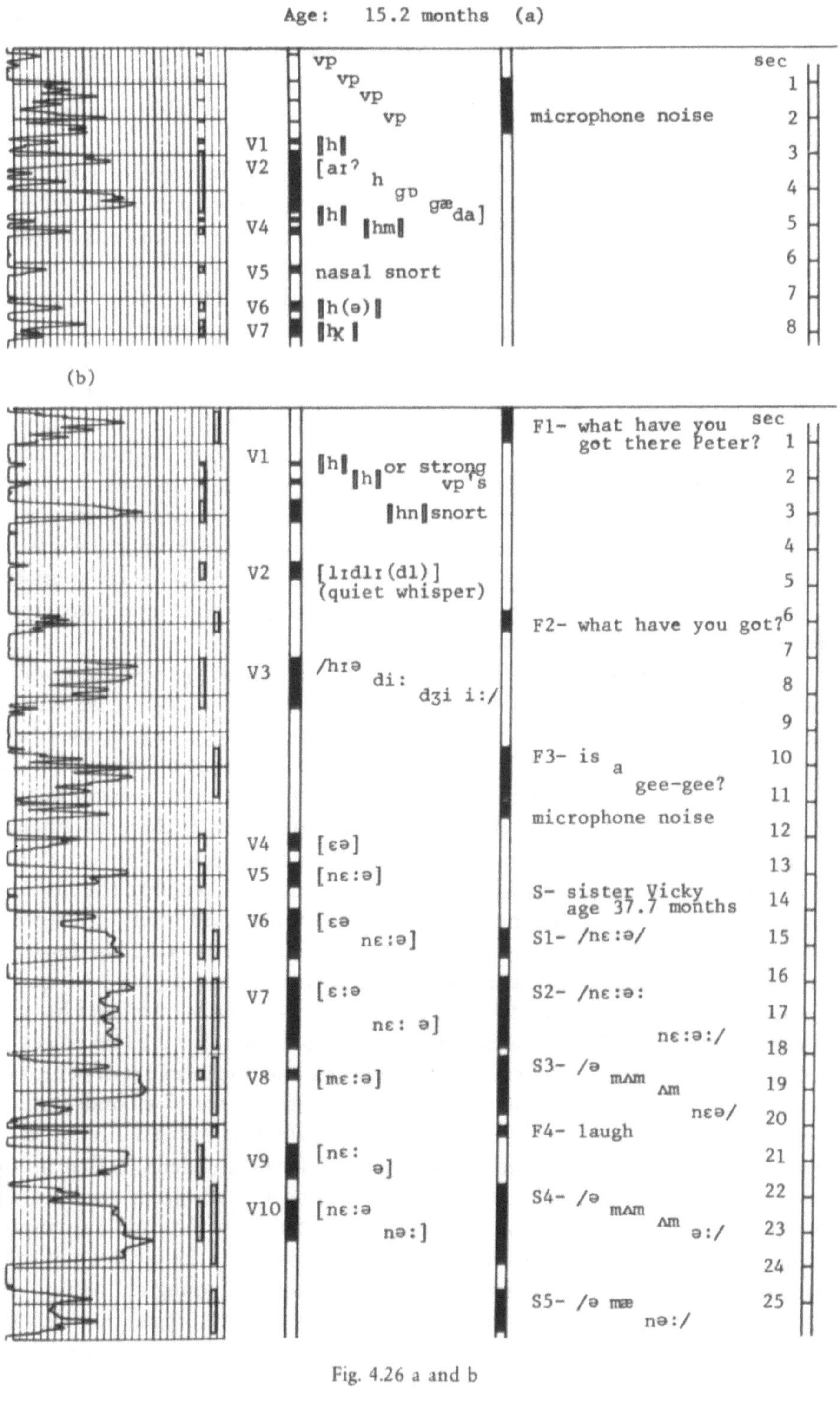

Fig. 4.26 a and b

delay, particularly if it is the culturally accepted norm, enhanced by doctors and others responsible for child care services, that baby noises are, quite simply, noises and not to be taken seriously. If the mother is conditioned into believing this vocal behaviour is unimportant, she will not give it the attention it deserves, in the face of all the many demands on her time of looking after the other children, running the home, and perhaps going out to work herself.

In the build-up to the vocalization V.3, a transient fragment of jargon was noted. It would appear that the child ascended through two demonstrable levels of complexity of organization of vocal behaviour before achieving his spoken words. There is the most primitive level of vocal pulsing, probably closely related to vocal panting behaviour, represented by "h" ... "h"; and there is the level of jargon, in which there is a high degree of organization of the vocal carrier wave but no linguistic content. These behaviours explain a universal feature of adult speech behaviour, especially if there is an element of uncertainty, tension or apprehension. The speech is punctuated by a series of brief vocal pulses of the "er" and "hm" variety in exactly the way that this 15 month-old child is behaving. One comes across jargon in adult speech (in the developmental sense of that word) only rarely. An example heard during the time span of writing this chapter was when someone was about to verbalize a comment but saw the partial negation of what she was just about to say, and which she had to modify in consequence. To her consternation and the listener's amusement the vocal result was a brief two pulses of pure jargon, identical in type with that shown at (b), V.2.

The remainder of (b) is interesting for light it throws on the ability of the younger child to adapt her vocal behaviour to that of a still younger child. Without taking any notice of the father's comment at F.3, the child begins a vocal play on the first vowel sounds of V.4, [ɛə]. No sooner had he produced [ɛə nɛːə] than his sister (S) joins in in precise imitation, soon changes her utterance to /əmʌmʌm/ but does not succeed in getting him to change his vocal pattern other than marginally.

In (c.i) a similar interaction took place 40 seconds later. The same sister, (Vicky aged 37.7 M) announces at (S.1) "I'm going to slide down onto the cushions" and as she does so the child, once again after an initial pulsed "h(er)" effort-sound utters a recognizable attempt, in tonal contour and segmentally, at "up down", an utterance which commonly accompanies such forms of physical play. He quickly repeats this, achieving a slightly more nasal quality on the "down" and his sister parodies him so well that it is almost impossible to distinguish the two voices. He then joins in the play with a great deal of chuckling and one moment of panic as he teeters uncertainly at the top of the settee. Play continues for 47 seconds until the next utterance is heard. This is seen in (c.ii) at V.1, which is the best attempt at "up down" heard so far. The father imitates him, the first time incidentally that another person, child or adult, had said "up down" during the whole of the recording session, confirming the spontaneity and appropriateness of the child's attempts at characterizing the play in word form. The child joins in for the second half of the utterance V.2, another characteristic verbal behaviour of young children.

The appearance of words, and the beginnings of truly linguistic behaviour, implies that from now on children will progressively model their segmental speech sounds on those used by their parents and others around them. It will be several

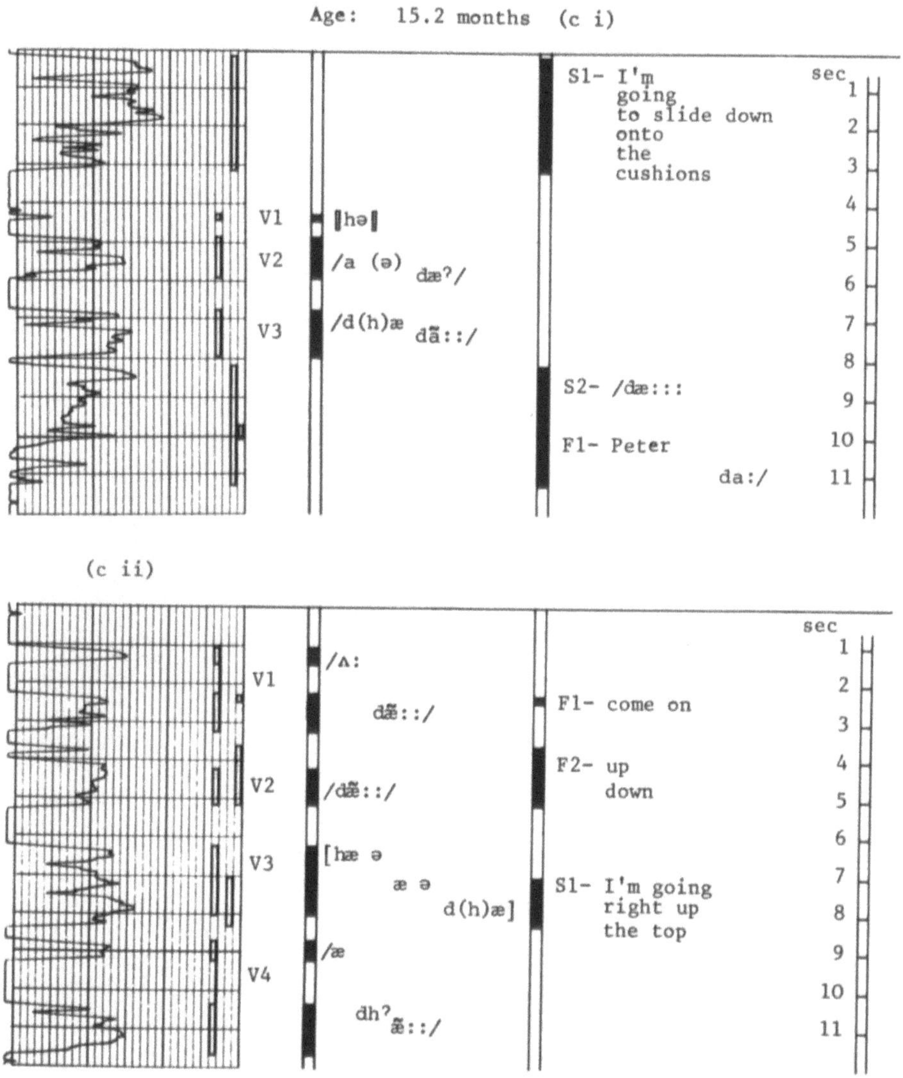

Fig. 4.26 c.i and ii

years before the full range of phonemes characteristic of the particular spoken language will be produced accurately as and when required in consecutive speech. We have seen that there are in effect three stages of development. There are the early vocal attempts of the child which produce "segmental" sounds in certain situations, related initially to the innate functioning of the neuromotor components of the vocal apparatus. These sounds were referred to as phonants. They were followed by, and overlapped with, segmental sounds which were considered to be modelled on adult speech sounds, but in which there was no unequivocal linguistic content. These phonals, as they were labelled for convenience, were limited in range, extent and precision and never amounted to more than a fraction of the repertoire of sounds required for normal spoken language. It seems likely that phonals are produced in a way which is essentially similar to that of the mature language speaker. The notion has already been discounted that we can as yet speak with any confidence about the manner of production of phonants.

We are then in a position to refute the long-standing assertion that the child in his first year of life produces all the sounds of the world's languages. Quite apart from its extraordinary neurodevelopmental implications, one can find no evidence for such a belief, which has something of that mystical quality which confuses so much thinking about language. If it is modified to the assertion that the new-born child is potentially capable of producing all the sounds of the world's languages, one could not argue, but the assertion then becomes so trivial that it is not worth stating. This alchemic search for the universal is a recurring preoccupation for the psycholinguist and one which runs counter to all other scientific disciplines whose base substance is human biology. Innumerable anatomical, physiological and cognitive features are universal; these are taken for granted since they are subsumed in the prefix "human". For those whose work is with the pathology of the human state it is the presence and extent of normal variation and the existence of anomalies which is highly significant, whether it be the surgeon carrying out an operation near some vital but possibly abnormally formed structure, or in the process of unravelling some complex disorder of language acquisition.

20. Peter 16.8 M

a) The child is looking at a book and his father has been patiently trying to get him to say "duck" without success, and then the two are diverted by a picture of a chicken. He returns to the previous picture and spontaneously produces V.1 in which the word "duck" is unmistakable, even to the faint but definite "k" at the end. The demonstrative word or phrase /iː jə/ is not so easy: it could be "here" though the double syllable structure makes this unlikely, or it could be a contraction of "(h)e(re) y(ou) are", an expression frequently used with children. There is the delighted approval of the father, more apparent in the exaggerated tonal contour than in the form of his words, with consequent repetition of the child's and father's comments at V.3 and F.3. After this the father continues with a "where" type question and subsequently modifies this to "show me" and the child obliges, uttering /dæ dʌʔ/, possibly repeating the form of his father's approval at F.1—"tha(t's a) duck".

b) A little later they are looking at another picture. Six seconds previous to F.1 the father had asked "Is it a choo-choo train" with no response, and he repeats the question in shortened form at F.1. After an interval of 7 seconds the child repeats his father's question-comment surprisingly precisely at V.2, and follows this in a very much quieter and more hesitant manner with "doo doo d(r) ai(n)". The manner of his speech implies considerable cognitive effort; he is probably recalling the father's original question-comment some 14—15 seconds earlier, and this delay and the length of utterance require a good deal of effort on his part. He has effectively signalled his intention to produce something by the indeterminate [æ̃] phonal, and this stops his father saying anything more after F.1 until the utterance has appeared. Oblivious of the immensity of his effort his father is unfeeling enough at F.2 to chide him gently on his pronounciation of the affricate /ʧ/ or "ch", which he had in fact managed surprisingly well as /d(ʒ)/ initially. Fortunately the child is quite undeterred, repeats "doo doo" with great pleasure and now finishes it off with the sound of a train whistle, as if to prove the extent of his accomplishment.

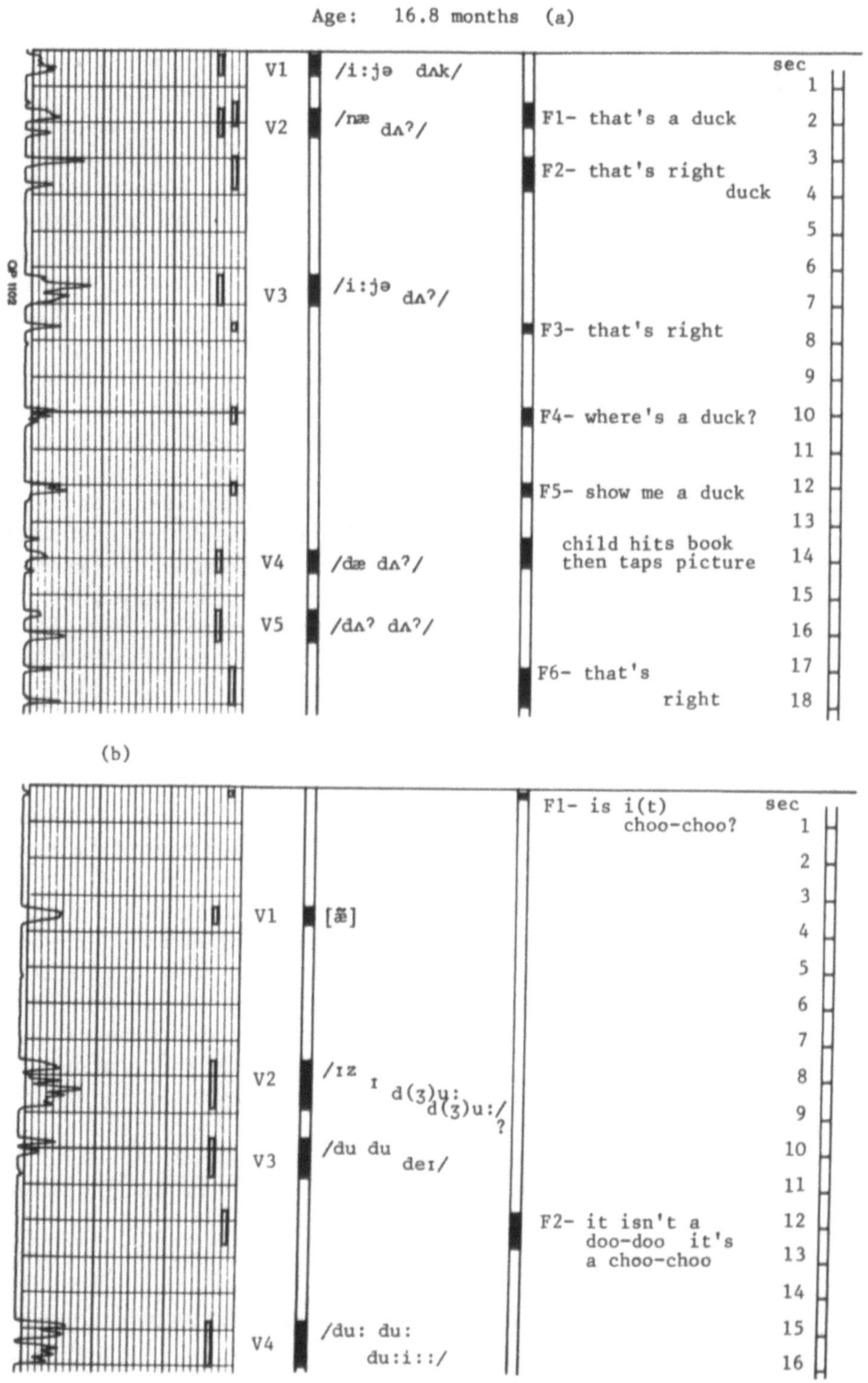

Fig. 4.27 a and b

21. Peter 18.6 M

The extent of verbal interaction and the communicative quality of which the child is capable continue to expand. His father has given him a book to look at (F.1) which he clearly disapproves of as a choice, pushing the book around and accompanying this activity at V.1 with some vocal complaint, the significance of which is clear though structurally it is a succession of phonals. His father finds the wanted book and his "This one alright?" meets with an approving "m" which his father imitates and then at V.4 the child gently and carefully produces "Thankyou" which is surprisingly accurate and socially appropriate. In passing it is worth noting the number of inaccuracies adults use when talking. In the transcriptions which have been figured on these pages there are a variety of grammatical errors in the parents' speech and F.4 is a case in point; his tag question, a linguistic device which takes a complex form in English, does not agree with the initial verb and should have appeared as "haven't you?". There then appears a very deliberately articulated six-syllable utterance. It is totally different in quality from jargon, the pulses of vocal energy occurring at the rate of 1.8 per sec and the phonemes at 5 per sec, and only one syllable is repeated. It is clearly linguistic in intention and overall structure though the precise details are obscure. It is obviously a spontaneously generated comment, and sounds as if there should be at least three and possibly four verbal elements in it. This is supported by the complex stress structure, which is also curiously difficult to be certain of—S (0 2 1 2 1 0). It is readily apparent that the perceptual quality of stress is not directly equivalent to loudness, which from the figure can be seen to increase in the first three and diminish for the last three syllables. The father understands the utterance sufficiently to accept it and comment appropriately on it.

It is instructive to compare the utterances which are beginning to appear in slowly increasing numbers from about twelve months on with those of the section at fourteen months. We have seen the vocal dexterity achieved by children in the production of tightly organized, compact and rapidly flowing pulses of sound characterized as jargon. This stage represents the height of achievement in the organization and control of the vocal carrier wave. Its successive phases have been followed from the innately determined vocal behaviour of the neonate; through the prolonged vocants with their marked pitch contours and medial closants, the first evidence of which was detectable at 0.9 M, and perfected in the activity of the 4.5 M child; then the progressive refinement of control, with the appearance of less florid vocal pulsing, the incorporation of an increasing number of phonal sounds and a more complex VCVCV structure; until the prolonged vocalizations described at 14.0 M with numerous pulses of sound, and the ability to vary the place and manner of production of consonantals.

Before this level of achievement in the control of the vocal carrier wave is fully perfected, another phenomenon begins to appear. Short utterances which are identifiable as words are produced from about 12.0 M. Though very simple in their vocal and segmental construction, they reveal a step-wise jump in complexity at the cognitive level. Even six months later the child is only able to produce 4—6 syllables in an utterance and this reveals something of the intellectual demand the activity

Age: 18.6 months

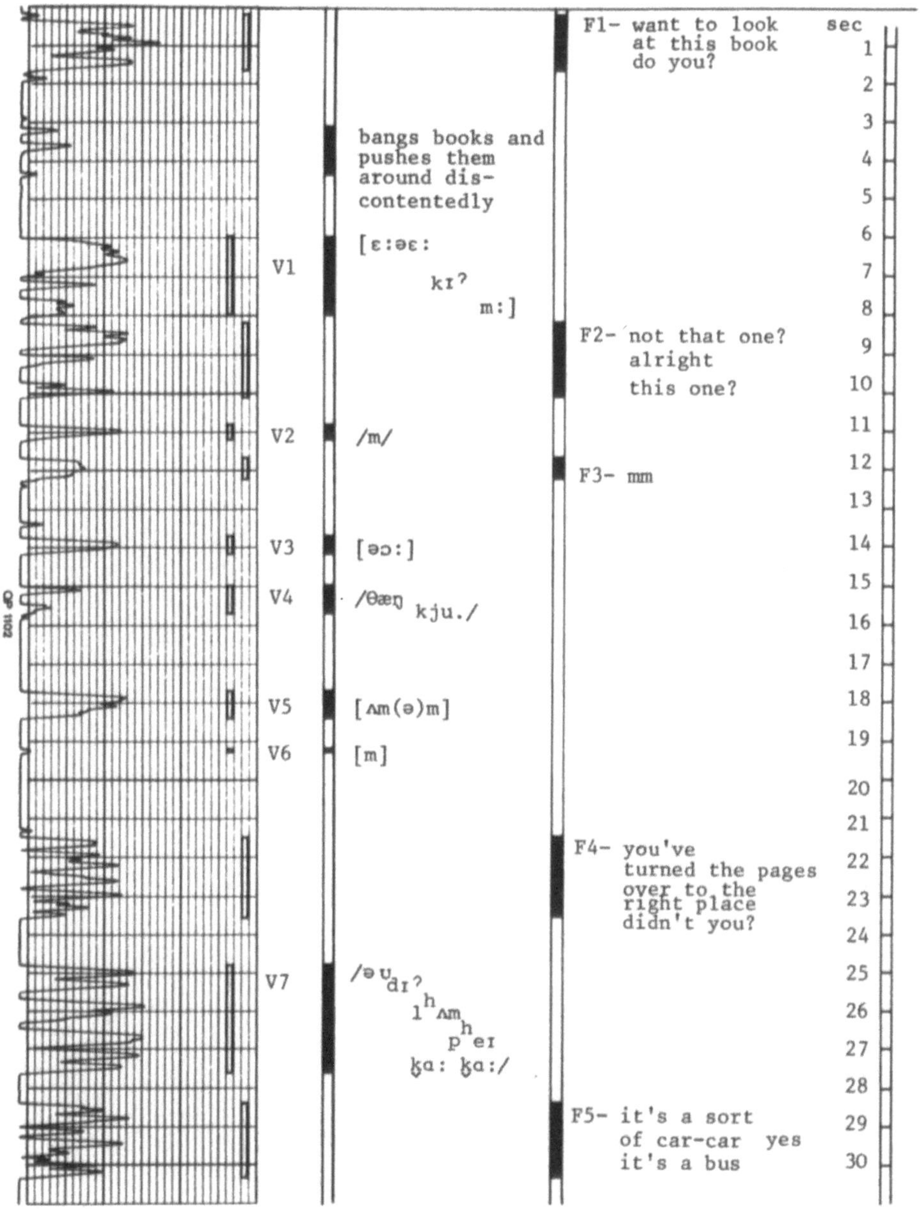

Fig. 4.28

makes on him. At 14.0 M he was capable, at the vocal level, of producing more pulses and phonals, and both of these features at a higher rate, than he demonstrates in this section. The recorded material shows evidence for even higher rates of production for these features of jargon after the age of 14 months which have not been included.

At first sight there appears to be a continous development of sound production from early infancy through the various stages of vocalization until fluent speech is achieved. The evidence obliges one to conclude that this concept is far from providing an accurate summary of child language development. The smooth transition that normally takes place during the second year of life from a vocal to a vocal-linguistic form of expression should not obscure the essential discontinuity between the ability to vocalize and the ability to talk. The conclusion gains further support from consideration of the problems of children with delayed or defective expressive language. To anticipate a later chapter, children are seen clinically in whom either the speech carrier wave or linguistic production (and often both) is at fault. This implies the necessity for discrete neurovocal and neurolinguistic mechanisms, even though the two normally function apparently as one.

22. Peter 20.0 M

Fig. 4.29 continues the theme of the previous section. The child's ability to understand language and to formulate its expression is further developed, and the examples given indicate the wide range of behaviours and his increasing mastery of the use of speech. He demonstrates at the same time his increasing cognitive development.

a) His opening comments refer to something which has fallen on the floor just before. He calls his father's attention to the fact with his "loo(k)" to direct attention so that the two will share the event, reinforcing the communitive ambiance. He returns to the book they are looking at and now, instead of resorting to vocal panting, exteriorizes his linguistic effort by a series of four utterances naming the boat until he is able to organize and utter the five-syllabled question about it at V.9. This is very similar in overall quality and form to the utterance in section 21, and in the same way gives the impression of a three- and possibly four-element sentence, though the precise details are not clear. He is probably asking where that boat has gone, after the page has turned over.

b) He has been given another book to look at, but perseverates with his label for the boat until he sees a tractor which he immediately names, and at V.14 once again invites his father to share the experience with him, who accordingly looks and makes an appropriate comment. The child for no readily discernible reason then recalls the earlier event in which a book fell on the floor, and echoes part of his father's comment at that time, saying "bu(m)p bumper no" in a worried voice, introducing a negative form and presumably wanting this book not to fall bump (on the floor).

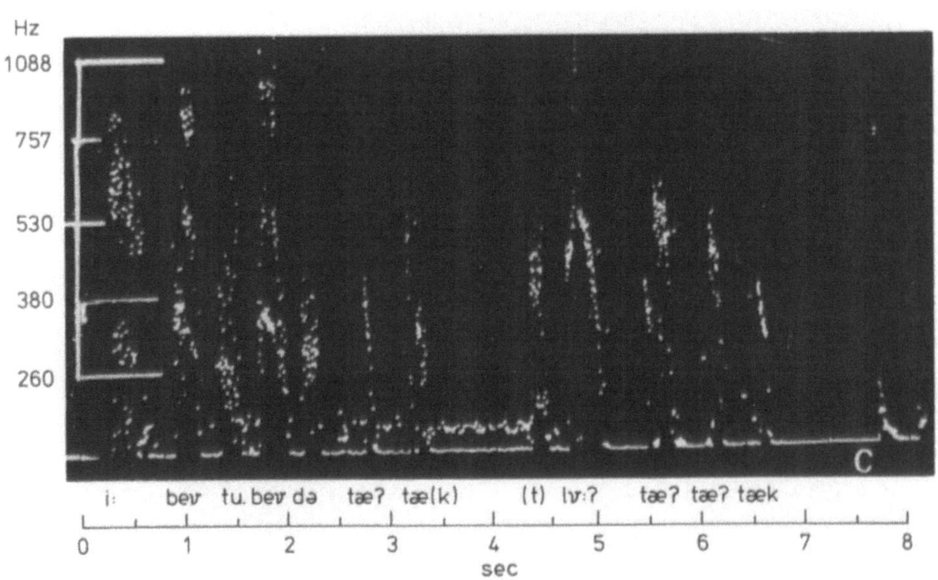

Fig. 4.30. Vocal pitch. Age 20.0 M; pitch changes accompanying animated communication, showing emphatic, discontinuous contours for each syllable in the utterances V.10—V.15 shown in Fig. 4.29 b

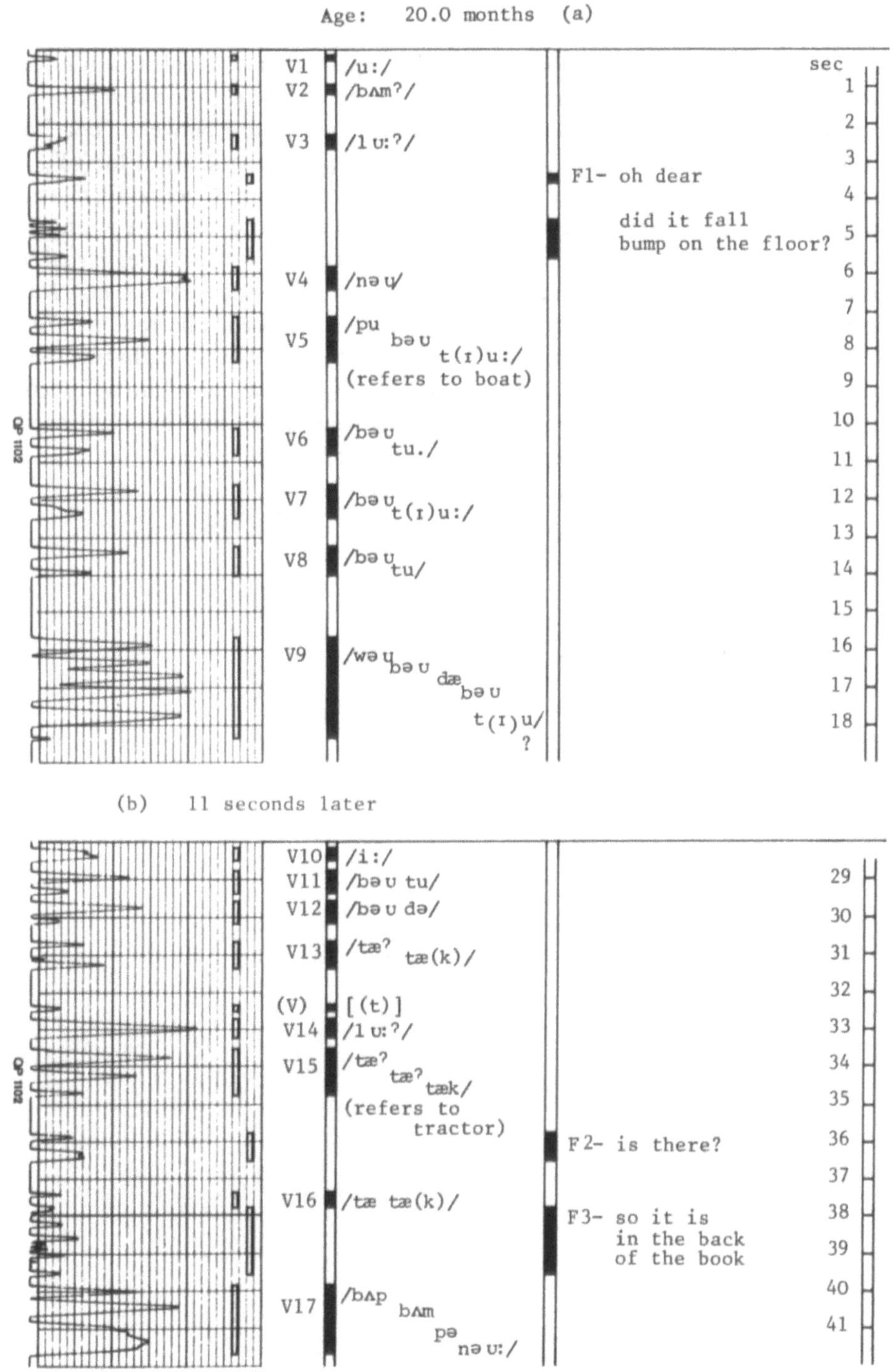

Fig. 4.29 a and b

c) He returns to the boat theme, enjoining the attention of both father and now mother also, who since they are discussing his use of the word "boat" fail to take any notice until his loud, peremptory "look". The father however wants him to show his mother something inside the book and clearly expects that he is able to understand the request, and the subsequent one to open the book. The child perseverates with "boatie" and in so doing produces an interesting confusion between "boat" and "book" saying in partial imitation of his father "ope(n) boatie a(nd) loo(k)". The sentence closes on a very concerned note, not apparent from its verbal form; something is wrong and it transpires that he is trying to open the book the wrong way, from its spine edge, and so is unable to. The sequence ends with another verbal confusion, occurring for a different reason from the book/boat one. He has now found the tractor his father wanted, and then produces a concerned "oh dear" in V.7 very clearly which then causes him difficulty as he tries to put all his thought together to express "oh dear, dirty tactac (tractor)". The sounds of "dear" and "dir(ty)" become fused together, and this interrupts his verbal flow since he realizes he is getting into difficulties, as shown by his repetitive, preliminary "oh oh oh ..."

(c) 1 min 40 sec after end of (b)

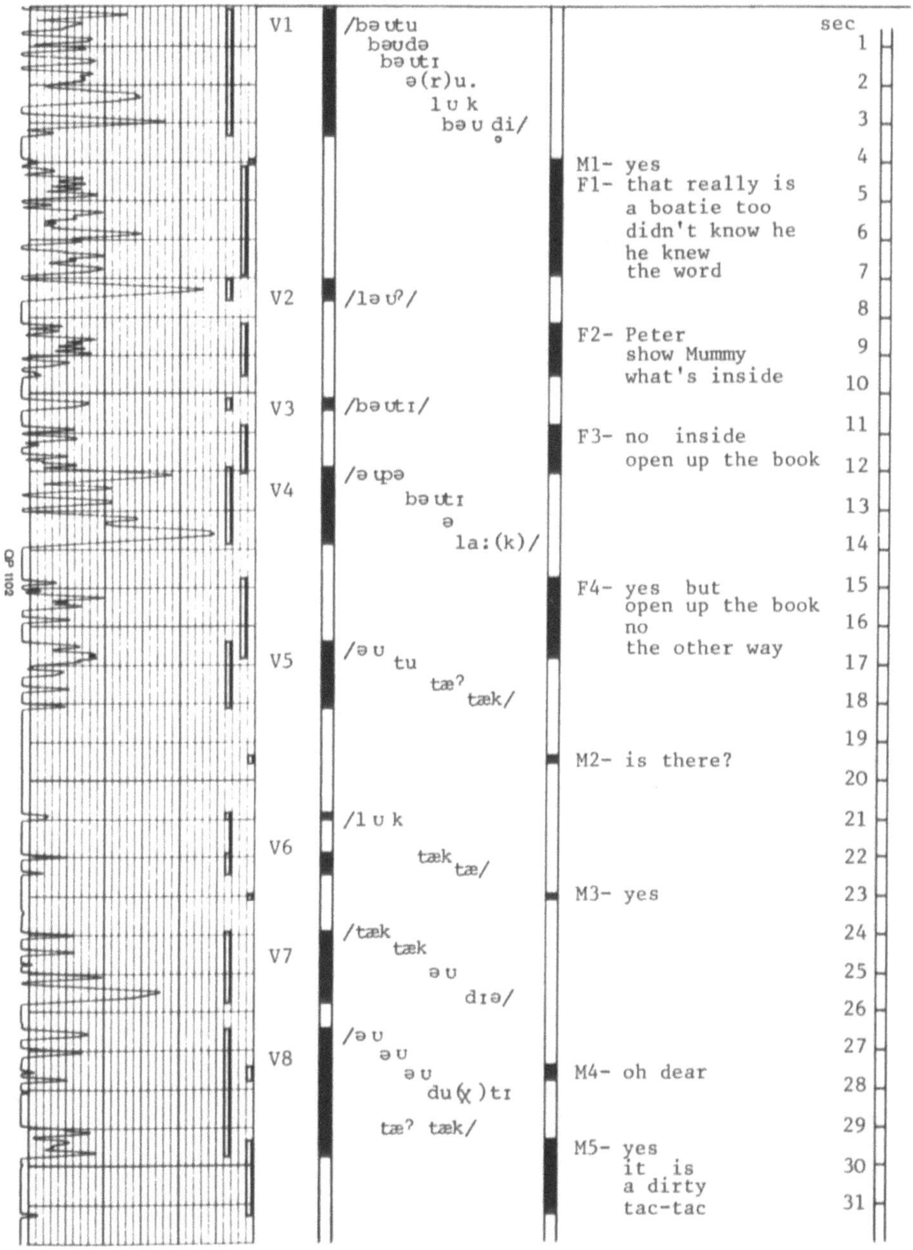

Fig. 4.29 c

d) In this final sequence his father asks him if he is playing with the tape recorder; his initial response is an affirmative "mm" to the question form, but there is then a long silence as he processes the linguistic content of the question and discovers to his consternation that he has given the wrong answer, since he shouldn't have been playing with it but in fact was! Hence the wary (and dishonest) "no". The situation is saved by the fortuitous appearance of the pet cat which he immediately notices and calls repeatedly, quickly changing back to the boat theme once again. After an "oh look" with the book in his grasp his pleasure turns to concern because once again there is something wrong. On this occasion he can see the boat but the book is round the wrong way. The sequence closes with him verbalizing his concern over the microphone being knocked over as he turns the book round.

In a short space of time he has observed a number of events and made a verbal comment on each as they arise; has expressed pleasure, concern, distress, prevarication; and has constantly been at work to maintain and deepen the level of communitive interaction with his parents.

Fig. 4.29 d →

(d) 36 sec after end of (c)

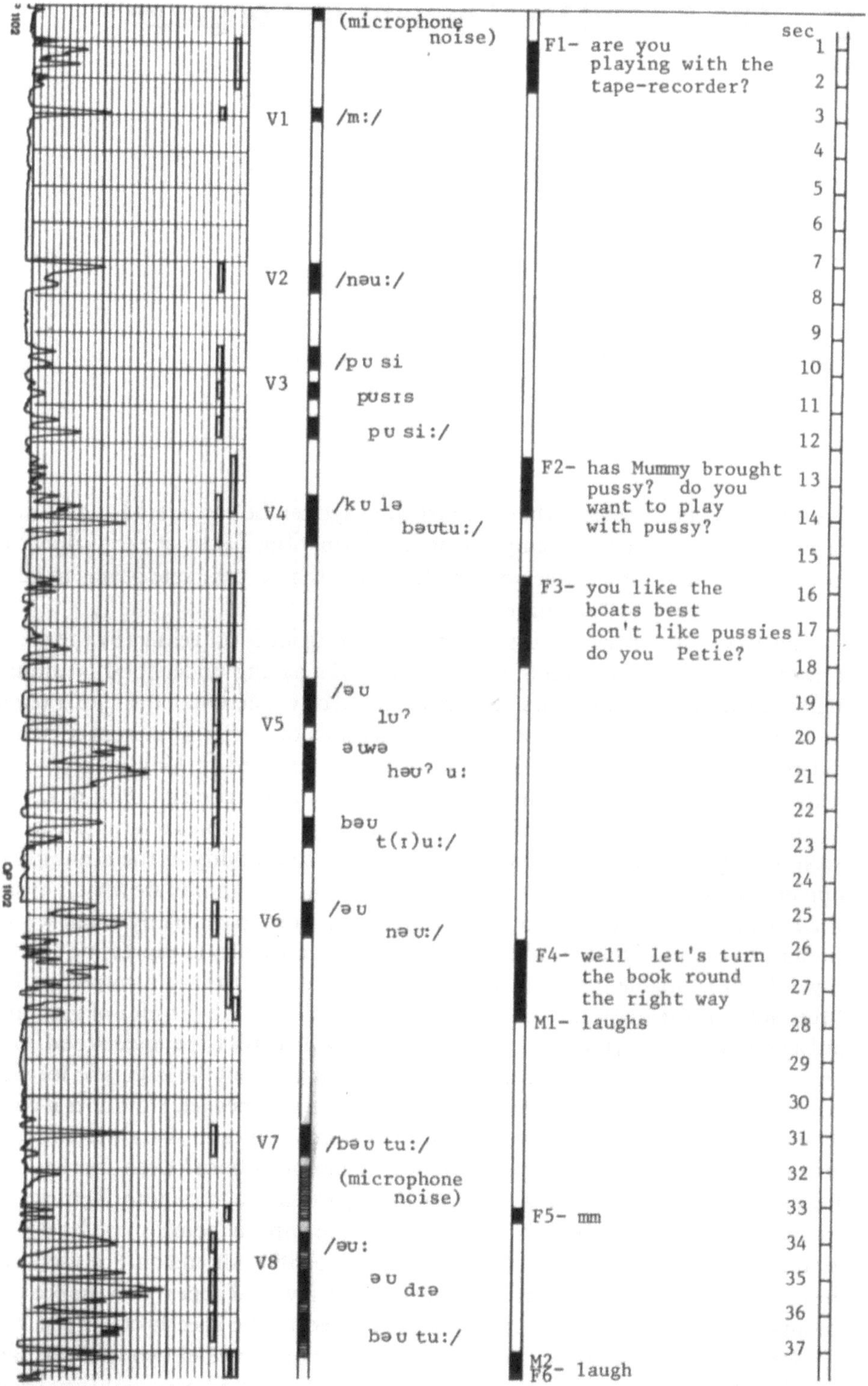

5 The Early Development of Language

The stage has been reached when spoken language can be considered and its early stages traced to the level of simple sentence formation. Taken at face value, this should not present too complex or lengthy a task, that is, until one begins to question what is meant by "language".

Language: a systematic means of communicating ideas or feelings by the use of conventionalized signs, sounds, gestures or marks having understood meanings; audible, articulate, meaningful sound as produced by the action of the vocal organs; the words, their pronounciation, and the methods of combining them used and understood by a considerable community and established by long usage; (rearranged from Webster's Third New International Dictionary, 1971, p. 1270).

In spoken language, the only form of language to be considered here, words are clearly paramount and words are such a basic commodity in the economy of human intercourse that no definition is needed in order to appreciate what is meant when "word" is referred to. But what in fact is a word, particularly when we are listening to a young child, or when a child has some difficulty in expressing himself in words, or is unable to articulate the sound pattern of the word correctly? The three facets of the definition of language quoted all include the idea of meaning, and it goes without saying that a vocal utterance which fails to be understood is not language, providing that certain assumptions are made about the linguistic, intellectual and other connections between the listener and the speaker. How does it come about that the child who has not yet uttered words comes to share the linguistic conventions of the community into which he has been born? Even more fundamentally, how does the child come to use these particular audio-motor signs we call spoken words in a way which indicates that meaning is being shared between speaker and listener? Though such a word as "impossible" should only be used with the greatest caution, and preferably not even then, it would appear to be impossible for any child to learn to talk unless he is exposed to the speech of others.

What are the rules which govern the interaction between two speakers, and especially between the competent adult and the little child who has only just begun to talk? It was because of the awesome complexity of the task faced by the child in learning language that some linguists were driven to postulate the existence of an innate "Language Acquisition Device". Chomsky formulated the components of such an acquisition model:

"A child who is capable of language learning must have
(i) a technique for representing input signals
(ii) a way of representing structural information about these signals
(iii) some initial delimitation of a class of possible hypotheses about language structure
(iv) a method of determining what each such hypothesis implies with respect to each sentence
(v) a method for selecting one of the (presumably, infinitely many) hypotheses that are allowed by (iii) and are compatible with the given primary linguistic data."

(Chomsky, 1965, p. 30)

In discussing how a child understands spoken language he goes on to say: "Thus what is maintained, presumably, is that the child has an innate theory of potential structural descriptions that is sufficiently rich and fully developed so that he is able to determine, from a real situation in which a signal occurs, which structural descriptions may be appropriate to this signal, and also that he is able to do this in part in advance of any assumption as to the linguistic structure of this signal."

(ibid., p. 32)

If one were considering the child from the point of view of adult language such a conclusion seems almost inevitable, and it is easy to sympathize with such a view. There is an element of truth in it, in that all human beings normally acquire spoken language. But so there is in the homunculus theory of human intra-uterine development, in which it was held that either in ovum or spermatozoon there was a perfect, preformed microscopic replica of the adult. In a conceptual sense there is. The advent of the microscope revealed the theory to be quite untenable in practice. The processes of mammalian embryogenesis and the processes of language development each depend on the emergence and progressive differentiation and organization of structures, cellular in the one, cognitive and communitive in the other.

The format of the description which follows is based on the words and word combinations which a child characteristically utters in the period between the first and third birthdays. It is important to remember that language, and language acquisition, is not purely linguistic. Cognitive function, the interaction between mother and child, and the relevant aspects of auditory processing and motor performance need constantly to be borne in mind, both for the normal development of language in the child, and in attempting to understand what happens when it is delayed or damaged. This multidisciplinary, panspecialist approach creates linguistic problems of its own: every field of knowledge has its own vocabulary and, what is more important but less obvious, its own traditions of converse and forms of enquiry. Much fruitless hypothesis formation and subsequent debate would be avoided if it were realized that though English speakers share a common tongue, we frequently do not speak the same language. Linguists and paediatricians, psychologists and physicists, speech therapists, teachers and parents each think and talk in different ways, with vastly different perceptions of the child.

The One Word Utterance

There are a number of ways of characterizing the language development of the child. One method widely used by developmental linguists is that of the "mean length of utterance" or MLU, proposed by Brown (1973). Because of the variation of verbal expression at any one age, he found it necessary to be able to compare the use of question forms, negatives and other aspects of syntactic structure after suitable readjustment made on the basis of a child's use of language. There is no easy answer to this problem. What a child says, and the way he says it, is dependent on many factors relating to the state of the child, the person who is talking to him, the relationship between them and the content of the discussion or nature of the play. A major obstacle in the use of MLU is that one cannot enter into meaningful discussion with the mother about the number of morphemes her child uses in an average utterance, so that one is drastically limiting the amount of information available. This may not matter to the researcher, but is an essential consideration for the clinician. Crystal, Fletcher, and Garman (1976) propose the adoption of a simple staging system based on the number of words a child produces in his utterances. It is an oversimplification to describe their approach quite in this way, particularly from the fourth stage on, but the rule holds well in the earlier stages. Stage I denotes the period during which the child uses one-word utterances, Stage II the production of two-word (strictly speaking "element" rather than "word") utterances, and so on up to and including Stage IV. These stages cover the chronological age of the child in six-month periods from the first birthday to the third, and it will be readily appreciated that the approach is simple in concept, and convenient in use.

A child's first words become recognizable to his parents at about the time of the first birthday. That some of these vocalizations really are words is highly debateable, and parents when questioned closely agree that "dad-dad" does not mean "daddy". It raises once again the question of what exactly is a word, and once again it is necessary to refer to the background and the purposes of the questioner. One's own approach, coloured by the clinical problems of children with severe hearing loss, or equally severe deficits in the neuromotor control of the speech apparatus, is to accept any stereotyped sound, used purposefully and which appears to have meaning, even if the parents are themselves not necessarily sure about the precise meaning until some time later. There is a definite difference in quality between a flow of babble or jargon-like sound and the deliberate utterance of a brief consonant-vowel(-consonant) "word".

In some children there can be no doubt that clearly spoken words are uttered long before the first birthday, and the parents (uncommonly but unequivocally) can provide a list of several words. In the majority these words are direct imitations of what has just been said to the child, and cannot be accepted within the limits of Webster's definition unless there is clear evidence of meaning for the child. Mimicry, and the long-deferred mimicry of the parrot, cannot be classed as language production unless there is additional clear evidence of purpose and comprehension, even though the "speech" of parrots is uncannily appropriate at times. Certainly by 14 months the average child has begun to use single words spontaneously and appropriately, and a month later speaks 2—6 words or more (Sheridan,

1975). The figures for growth of vocabulary are rather variable so that at one extreme Sheridan gives a cautious estimate of 50 or more words, whilst M. E. Smith (1926) gives the surprisingly high figure of 272, at the second birthday. The differing professional backgrounds of these two women, the one clinical the other academic, must influence such figures. The majority of children will probably have a vocabulary size between the two, of perhaps 100—200 words. In round terms the figures at the third birthday given by Smith are 900 words, and at the fourth and fifth, 1500 and 2000 words respectively. If one considers the rate of vocabulary increase it is possible to derive from the data reported by Smith the number of new words which a child will use on average in a week. At 15 months this will be 1—2 words, increasing to about 7 words from 21—30 months, and rising to a peak of 17 new words in a week at the third birthday, after which it falls to 12 words and continues at this level until the age of five is reached when there is a further slight fall to 8—10 words.

The advent of words is a highly significant stage in human development. It may be summarized briefly by saying that the child has completed an astonishingly complex transformation from perceiving and identifying some visual (say) stimulus as coming from a particular type or class of object, developing and retaining an internal and permanent representation of that object, and giving this internalized image of objective reality a label. This label bears no conceivable resemblance to the object, unlike a symbol in which there is some residual element of representation which maps onto the original object, whether it be a miniaturized model car or animal, or a picture, or more remotely, in the drawing of a matchstick man. Words are signs, stereotyped conventions, and as such cannot be understood outside the community in which they are used. Before the child acquires the use of these signs he is obliged to show that he understands the meaning or significance of a particular object by an appropriate behaviour. He will for instance hold the spoon or the cup the proper way, or will pick up a hairbrush and brush his hair with it, demonstrating his knowledge of its use. Once the cup or brush has a label this is no longer necessary, and he can refer to the object by name. The name encapsulates not only the object as a discrete entity, but other aspects also, such as its function or use.

The Meanings of Words

When a child uses a label in this way, what exactly is he doing? When he sees a dog, he may say "Dog" or some other word which his parents accept as his label for it, but to what is he specifically referring? In asking this question, E. V. Clark (1974) points out that he may be referring to one of many features which characterize it, such as being four-legged, or it might be his coat, his movement or his bark. The child will of necessity rely on a limited number of features to identify it, including the shape and size, the sound, the texture or the pattern of activity. The result is that the child will have an understanding of the word "dog" which may only partially overlap with the adult use of the word. As Moerk (1977) puts it, the child's concept and the adult's are not equivalent for some time. The meaning, or semantic space occupied by a concept, is not clearly delimited until there has been considerable redefinition arising out of the child's experience of it in use, ultimately converging on the generally accepted usage of his immediate community. Until that time the child will use words in a variety of inappropriate ways.

Over-extension describes the child's usage of words in which generalization has been carried too far, so that for instance "doggie" refers to cats, cows and horses and any other four-legged animal as well as dogs. "Dadda" may not be used to refer to the one specific person, but to all males, though usually there are certain limits to the child's misconception. Clark (1974) has found that this type of labelling is especially prominent during the time from 1 y 1 m—2 y 6 m and rarely lasts for longer than a year in any one child. She hypothesizes that a word is used to refer to some perceptually salient characteristic of an object, and so is used for all such occurrences of the characteristic, until with increasing experience this is found not to be correct. As this negative feedback builds up, so the child begins to realize that his use of a word and that of his parents is different and a noticeable change in verbal behaviour takes place. By the end of this period of over-generalization the child is constantly (parents might say incessantly, even voraciously) asking questions of the "What?" type, and this coincides with the very high rate of vocabulary growth noted already. The reverse type of error occurs and the child uses a word as if it were a name rather than a label, so that only one particular boy is "Boy". Such over-specificity may be seen in other behaviours during the second year, the child refusing to drink out of any mug or cup except his one special one, and certain activities must be carried out in unvarying, precisely ordered ways.

These errors of generalization help to reveal the importance of the principle of generalization in language acquisition. Moerk (1977) points out that the child with his limited vocabulary is in a sense obliged to apply one general term to a large variety of objects; the smaller the vocabulary, the broader the range of concepts which have to be labelled with the same word. There is not a great deal of information available on the relationship between the child's ability to categorize objects and events cognitively and the verbal labels he uses for them. Words are used to refer to objects as wholes, and it is only later that particular properties or features can be alluded to. Similarly the child can only label the essential characteristics of certain states, conditions or activities (Menyuk, 1971) using words like "gone" or "broken".

It is highly probable that the child will have a series of rules about the way he will use the words in his limited vocabulary for maximum effectiveness. Greenfield (1978) considers that the child follows a rule of informativeness. "What, from the child's point of view, can be assumed is not stated; what cannot be assumed or taken for granted is given verbal expression by the single word." In an example, her son Matthew says "car" when he hears a car going past outside the window, or when he is pointing to his own toy car which is not actually in his hand. In these instances he is referring to something which is relatively uncertain since the one could not be seen, and the other was not being held; by saying "car" he conveys the maximum amount of information. Once he has the car in his hand its existence is certain; there is no need to refer primarily to it, and he refers to some other aspect of the car, depending on what is happening. As he pushes it he says "bye bye", and when he has thrown it down he says "down". Now that the car is no longer in his possession, it is not the change of state of the car he refers to, but the object itself and he says "car" again. There is a continual shift of reference depending on what can be assumed and what, in being expressed, gives the most information.

The Holophrase

When a child uses a word, it may not be possible to decide on the precise significance or purpose of the utterance, certainly on linguistic grounds alone. With this uncertainty in mind it is clearly possible for the adult listener to ascribe to the child a variety of intentions in speaking, and to his utterance a variety of meanings. Single word speech is often called "holophrastic" in consequence. McNeill (1970) defines it as the possibility that the single word utterances of young children express complex ideas, and in giving the example "ball" points out that the child may not simply be naming such an object, but may want it, or want someone to look for it. He goes on: "Holophrastic speech means that while children are limited to uttering single words at the beginning of language acquisition, they are capable of conceiving something like full sentences." (ibid., p. 20)

The more extreme view of earlier writers such as Stern and Stern (1907) or Leopold (1949) and others is that the young child's single word utterances are equivalent to full adult sentences. This makes the child the miniature image of the adult, and conveys too much inexplicable "innateness". The term holophrase carries a heavy burden of theoretical implication. In developmental terms the child is only able to formulate simple sentences perhaps a year after his first words, and it is not for a further year or more after that that the complex sentences of more adult speech begin to appear. Cognitively, as we have seen, the child in his second year has only started on the task of unravelling the intricate causal relations which underlie the ideas of an agent acting on an object to produce an effect. It will be another six months to a year before the simplest verbal expression of this concept can be achieved. Rodgon (1976) uses the word slightly differently and less ambitiously when she says that "holophrase" refers to a single-word utterance which is used by a child to express more than the meaning usually attributed to that single word by adults. As we have seen, this may be true or not true in the sense that a child may over-generalize, under-generalize or even use several different words for the same object. These problems arise out of imperfectly developed verbal concepts, and even more so from the imprecise cognitive concepts underlying them. Piaget talks about the elaboration of the object concept at the age of 9—12 months, saying that it is possible the object is still not the same to the child as it is to us.

"Thus the object is, perhaps, to the child, only a particularly striking aspect of the total picture in which it is contained ... there would still exist only images such as 'ball-under-the-armchair' ... 'papa-at-his-window', etc." (Piaget, 1954, p. 62—63)

These are in effect "cognitive holophrases" in which the basic concepts are as yet undifferentiated; there is instead an amalgam of the object concept and its spatial location, both of which are themselves imperfectly defined. The situation for the child's single word utterances appearing somewhat later in time is almost identical. Of course the child is referring to more than he can say, but in the opposite sense or direction from which the users of the linguistic label "holophrase" picture the child's conceptual and linguistic abilities. There appears to be no developmental justification for the use of the term, and certainly, as Dore (1975) similarly asserts, no evidence that the child at the one-word stage has any notion of sentences. The difficult task of learning the syntax of his language, the different categories of words, the way in which these may be combined and the basic rules of word order so that phrases, clauses and sentences may be built up and spoken will occupy the child for a number of years in the future.

Speech Acts

Dore (1975) considers that the basic unit of communication using spoken language is the "speech act", and in the early, one-word stage the speech act has two components. These are the word used and the "force", typically defined by the intonation. "Mama" could appear with three different intonation patterns depending on whether the child was merely labelling his mother, or some doll as the mother; asking if an object belonged to his mother; and calling his mother to him from some distance. In this way Dore considers that the child is performing three different (primitive) speech acts—labelling, requesting and calling, which comprise the differing forces of the utterances. Examples of the full range of one-word or primitive speech acts in two children *M* and *J* reported by Dore is shown in Table 5.1.

Table 5.1. *Primitive speech acts*

Primitive speech act	Description of example
Labelling	M touches a doll's eyes, utters /aɪz/, then touches its nose, utters /noʊz/; she does not address her mother and her mother does not respond.
Repeating	M, while playing with a puzzle, overhears her mother's utterance of *doctor* (in a conversation with the teacher) and M utters /datə/; mother responds *Yes, that's right honey, doctor,* then continues her conversation; M resumes her play with the puzzle.
Answering	Mother points to a picture of a dog and asks J *What's this?;* J responds /ba wa /.
Requesting (action)	J tries to push a peg through a hole and when he cannot succeed he looks up at his mother, keeping his finger on the peg, and utters /ʌ ʌ ʌ / (with constant contours and minimal pause between syllables); his mother then helps him push the peg, saying *Okay.*
Requesting (answer)	M picks up a book, looks at her mother and utters /bʊk↑/ (where arrow indicates a rising terminal contour); mother responds *Right, it's a book.*
Calling	J, whose mother is across the room, shouts /mâma/ loudly (where ˆ indicates an abrupt rising-falling contour); his mother turns to him and says *I'm getting a cup of coffee. I'll be right there.*
Greeting	J utters /haɪ/ when teacher enters room; teacher responds *Hello.*
Protesting	J, when his mother attempts to put on his shoe, utters an extended scream of varying contours, while resisting her; M, in the same circumstance, utters *No.*
Practising	M utters *daddy* when he is not present; mother often does not respond.

Examples of primitive speech acts of two one-year-old children, M and J, from Dore (1975): J. Child Language 2.31.

The Nature and Purposes of Language

In a list such as that of Dore's, or for instance in the description of the emergence of the various types or purposes of utterance by Greenfield and Smith (1976), it is clear that the single word can be an astonishingly versatile tool. In the second year of life he is already able to use words in a wide variety of different ways, depending on his purpose, intention and needs at the time he speaks. There is in consequence a much greater interest now in these practical aspects of language so that "pragmatics" as it is called, is a serious branch of study, along with the syntax, semantics, and phonological aspects. Underlying the use of language, of which Dore's list provides a useful summary at this early stage, there would appear to be three primary, elemental functions. These may be labelled as communicative, cognitive and communitive, and they are already in evidence at this first stage of language development. Any speech activity which involves another person is clearly involving communication, and it would appear at times, and with some writers that language and communication are synonymous. Communication between persons is an essential feature of human behaviour and it would be superfluous to take the point further, but it is only part of the picture.

Cognitive activity. It is difficult to over-emphasize the importance of human intellectual activity, of perception and inference, as an essential antecedent to the spoken word. But this is not to say (and it may as well be said at this stage, from the time that the young child utters his first hesitant words) that words have no effect in their turn on the child's cognitive processes. Once such an exquisite tool became available, it would be profligate in the extreme not to make the fullest use possible of it. An interesting experiment by Sachs and Truswell (1978) reveals that children at the one-word stage are able to carry out purely verbal requests, requests which, in a sense, could not have been envisaged other than through the medium of words. Words are a remarkably succinct and economical way of summarizing the world in which we live, of ordering it and of making sense of it. This applies very much more to some features of the environment and of ourselves than to others: we are for instance remarkably inefficient at the adequate portrayal and communication of emotion. Words quite literally fail us, and we resort to banalities or take refuge in helpless silence. It is partly for this reason that non-verbal expression, art in its various forms and some sports also, is not marginal or frankly irrelevant, but is essential to a healthy well-ordered society—and perhaps even more so when it is otherwise.

Words help the child in the organization of his world, a process in which he is helped by his parents, as he learns the names of objects and of activities. Individual objects begin to be collected into sets or classes—things that are always associated with eating, such as a spoon, a plate, a beaker; or bedtime or bathtime. There is the process of natural association, which is extended enormously by the use of words, and at a faster rate than would otherwise be possible. Items can be grouped verbally, using a functional category such as things to eat with, or things that go on the road, though collective words like cutlery or vehicles will appear very much later. "Objects" can be living or inanimate, funny or frightening, strange or familiar, nice or nasty, boring or exciting and so a wide variety of possible ways of classifying the environment and the activities which are immediately relevant to the child begin to develop. The child builds up as it were his own theory of knowledge of the world, and words play a creative part in this, mediating and facilitating the cognitive processes by which it can take place.

Communitive activity. The communitive function of language can be identified in numerous verbal utterances, but in forms which are easily overlooked. Greetings form a universal feature of human meeting and there is in many languages an elaborate and extended ritual governing their use. A mother shows her own forms of ritual with her child however young, greeting him if she has only left him minutes before, or even during the same interaction if his attention has wandered off their "joint" involvement. Taking leave of someone is another example of the same process, and "hallo" and "bye bye" are some of the earliest words a child will learn. Words such as these, far from being unimportant, underlie and reinforce the fundamental human behaviour of being with another person, of joining her and leaving her. Much verbal activity can scarcely be classed as communicative, let alone as of any cognitive significance, often being mundane, repetitive and with no apparent underlying pattern or purpose. This may be intensely irritating to some individuals, who can see no point in such trivial forms of converse. Once it is realized that the talking is a tangible expression of the desire to be in another's company, to be with another, the activity is highly significant. The young child is adept at ensuring that some loved, familiar person is with him, and much of his speech activity is devoted to this end.

Interaction with Mother

The time which a child shares with his mother and other competent language speakers whose company he especially enjoys, provides the essential opportunity for him to learn to talk. We have seen in Chapter 4 many of the ways in which the very young child and his mother learn to attend jointly to some shared interest or activity. Bruner (1975) says that once attention is jointly directed, the mother will systematically act upon or comment upon what has caught their joint attention, though the process is not so one-sided as this might suggest. Snow (1977) considers that mothers talk with their children on the assumption that a conversational type of interaction is the most appropriate. This implies a reciprocal process in which the mother assumes she can communicate information to her child, and can in her turn receive information from him. In essence, the mother's speech is related to the child or his activities and his direction of attention, and much of it is directed towards eliciting responses from him. It will be seen from this that there is more to the acquisition of language than the specifically linguistic aspects. In Snow's view, as in Bruner's, there is the sharing of some common interest, a dynamic process involving the active participation of both mother and child; and the notion of turn-taking, in which the mother and the child constantly change roles, from being speaker to becoming the listener. A variety of devices are adopted to indicate the relinquishing of one's turn, or one's intention to retain it. They include facial expression and hand gesture, and the taking in of a breath, or its release. Non-verbal speech devices include the pattern of intonation and the stress and rhythm of the speech, the continuation of speaking, or the nature of the pause and its duration, whilst the use of the question format is a clear demonstration in words of the intention to hand the speaking mode to the listener.

The characteristics of the mother's speech reveal a number of modifications from that used with adults. Her utterances are shorter in sentence length, simpler in construction, and there is an increased amount of natural redundancy (Snow, 1977). This is also achieved through a more repetitive type of delivery. The pitch of the voice tends to be higher, and there is a definite exaggeration of the prosodic features of speech, with more clearly marked patterns of intonation. Pauses are clearly marked and there are numerous question forms. The content of her speech is related very much to the child, what he is looking at and what the two of them are doing. It is therefore rooted in the here and now, and there is in consequence a preponderant use of the present tense. Whilst all this is going on the mother is constantly monitoring her child's play and other activities, the level of his attention, the tempo and duration of their interaction and the quality of response she is gaining from him. This feedback from the child is quite essential. It is shown by his facial expression; the sense of enjoyment he is deriving from the joint activity; his vocal, verbal and non-linguistic responses; his readiness to take the turns offered him; and his own initiative in carrying on the interaction, even when his mother has indicated her intention of stopping, and attending to something else.

In an interesting and carefully controlled study reported by Ringler (1978), comparisons were made of the speech between adult-adult and adult-child, and in this latter group the differences were noted between the speech to children aged 10—13 months, and 22—25 months. The mean rate of speaking between adults was 61 words per minute, whilst it fell to 34 words per minute to the children, with a slower rate for the younger group. There was a trebling of the amount of speech to the children by their second birthdays. This was felt to be a reflection of the mother's awareness of the child's increased need for language stimulation, and of his increased ability to grasp the meaning of syntactically complex utterances. This is partly revealed in the data for length of utterance, which was less than two words to the one-year-olds, more than three words to the two-year-olds and 7—8 words between adults. The most frequent category of speech in this study was commands, to either age of child, and the relative frequency of questions increased for the older group, for whom there were only a small proportion of statement sentences; repetition had dropped substantially by this age. A further important conclusion of the study was a clear indication that the way a mother addresses her two-year-old may have lasting effects on speech and language development as measured at the age of five.

The style of interaction, and the nature of the language offered to the child and by him, has not yet received as much attention as it deserves. Lieven (1978) found a marked difference between the speech of the two children studied, and between that of their respective mothers. Both were 18 months old or a little more when the study started. One of the children talked slowly and coherently about the activities and objects in her environment, whilst the other girl devoted more time in trying to engage her mother's interest. The mother of the first child rarely failed to respond to her utterances, whilst the other failed to respond to over half of her daughter's, showed less interest in what she was saying and made less effort to keep the conversation going. It might appear that the differences in conversational style (though in the second mother-child pair the investigator considered that there was little evidence of conversation in the sense described by Snow) were due to the mother in each instance, but this would seem too simple an explanation, and the nature and personality of the child have an important part to play.

The Child's Understanding of the Spoken Word

The numerical size of the child's spoken vocabulary gives valuable information on the child's acquisition of language, providing that his age is also taken into consideration. To this needs to be added the types of words used and the ways in which the child uses them. This is not enough. The linguistic output of his utterances will inevitably give some indication of what the child can understand, at least by inference and in the child in whom language is developing normally. There needs in addition to be accurate information on what he is able to understand when others talk to him, such as can be provided by the Reynell Developmental Language Scale (Reynell, 1969). This has received very much less attention than his own spoken language, partly because it is much more straightforward a procedure to write down or record what the child says in the various situations in which he is being studied. There is of necessity a much greater level of direct involvement with the trained investigator, when the child's ability to carry out specific requests to demonstrate his comprehension is being measured in some way. Nevertheless, when one considers the small numbers of children usually included in studies of language development, and the fact that in many the investigator is one of his parents, it is surprising that there is not much more quantitative information available. As it is, the discussions which take place on the important relation between verbal expression and comprehension—a relation which is of crucial importance in clinical practice, are not notably well informed. The all-too-often repeated comment that comprehension is always ahead of expression lacks conviction, and it seems much more probable that there is no fixed, constant ratio between the two. At times and for certain stages in language development there may well be a considerable gap between the two, whilst at others it may be that there is no significant difference.

There is very little information available on the extent of the child's recognition vocabulary. Sheridan (1975) describes the 9-month-old as being able to react appropriately to one or two words; by the first birthday this has extended to several words in the right context, and he will carry out simple instructions like "Give it to Daddy" or "Clap hands". Parents describe a number of reactions to words during this three-month period; the child will look round for his sister when her name is said, or will search for "Pussy", will hold out his foot when some comment is made about his shoe, and so on. Children at the one word stage frequently give the impression that they are able to understand longer utterances. It is often the case that they are responding to a particular word which they recognize, especially when it is uttered in the course of a well-established routine, so that there is the additional structure of the situation to guide them. This is not always or necessarily the case. Sachs and Truswell (1978) were able to demonstrate in 12 children aged from 1 y 4 m–2 y 0 m who were only able to say single words, that they could carry out a range of requests in which it was essential for them to recognize both components of a two-word utterance. The requests were of the type "Kiss (or Tickle) Bunny (or Dolly)" and both elements of the request had to be complied with for a correct response to be scored. With a mean number of instructions to each child of 15.8, the number of correct responses was 9.2 (58%), the child being presented with four different possibilities of response to any one request. There were relatively few partially correct responses, a form of response which would indicate that the child had responded to only one of the two words in the utterance. Furthermore, some of the requests were completely novel, the child being asked to carry out some faintly ridiculous or unusual task, confirming that meaning was conveyed to the child by language alone.

Two and Three Word Utterances

An advance of fundamental importance takes place when the child is about 18 months old. He begins, in a halting and uncertain manner, to combine one word with another, and it is from this time on that the astonishing versatility of language begins to be revealed. Once the joining of one word to another has been accomplished the possibility arises of three, four and an ever increasing number of words being put together into a consecutive utterance. If utterances were restricted to two words in length and there were no rules about word combination, a modest vocabulary of 1000 words, achieved by children soon after their third birthday, could generate virtually a million two-word utterances. But by that age a child is already putting four and usually more words together. It is no wonder that this ability to generate combinations of words explains why some consider language really begins at this stage.

"In the sense that language is essentially a means for expressing an unlimited number of ideas with a limited system, this is the true beginning of language."

(Dale, 1976, p. 40)

It is a point of view with which one has a good deal of sympathy, and would be able to endorse if the child at the one-word stage was limited to labelling people and objects in his utterances. In Chapter 4 it was seen that this is not the case. Long before he has joined two words together he has used single words in a number of different ways, for a number of different purposes. If grammatical structure is considered a necessary component of language, then language cannot really be said to start before words are joined. The issue is not quite so theoretical as it seems at first sight. To anticipate aspects of disorder, clinical experience reveals that there are children who have difficulty in ascribing meaning to single words, and in using them meaningfully. This process, of deriving signs from symbols from items and events experienced in the objective world, is very different from the process in which, given a number of words in a vocabulary, the child starts combining them together. What appears to be a simply ordered process when viewed from one aspect may in fact be an expression of many different processes. To put it another way, the orderly sequence of one-word followed by two-word followed by three-word utterances is only the surface tip of a remarkably extensive, highly structured cognitive-linguistic iceberg.

The appearance of new two-word combinations was reported by Braine (1963) for one child to be fourteen in number one month after the first had appeared, and in the subsequent one-month periods—10, 30, 35, 261, 1050. This growth curve, with its very slow initial rate of increase, followed by a remarkable rate of increase in the later months is of a strictly logarithmic form. The increasing facility which the child shows in combining two words must be, in part at least, an expression of his mastery of the ways in which two words can be put together, and his greater understanding of the purpose and function of his utterances. This is not the straightforward matter it might appear and explanatory descriptions of the two-word stage are continually being modified.

Pivot grammars. Braine described the child's utterances as having two components. In one child studied, "bye bye" occurred in combination with 31 other words, always being the first of the two; similarly "see" was followed by 15 other words. Analyses of this type led him to propose a grammatical structure in which the words which recurred in first position in two-word combinations would be called "pivot" words, "since the bulk of the word combinations appear to be formed by using them as pivots to which other words are attached as required" (Braine, 1963). The pivot class of words was small in number and the complementary class was formed by the other words of which there were many and comprised the "X" class. Examples from this same child included: "see—boy/ sock/ hot"; "allgone—shoe/ vitamins/ egg"; "byebye—plane/ hot"; "pretty—boat/ fan"; "big—boat/ bus"; "my—mommy/ milk"; "hi—plane/ mommy". This form of analysis came to be widely used, though certain modifications were necessary. Braine, in the child for whom some examples have been quoted, also listed the instance of a pivot word which came second rather than first: "do—it", "push/ close/ move—it". McNeill renamed the "X" class, calling it the "open" class. He summarized the principles of the classification in the following way —

"When these analyses are conducted on speech collected from children of 18 months or so, at the very beginning of patterned speech, at least two classes of words emerge. One contains a small number of words, each frequently used—the 'pivot' class. The other contains many more words, each infrequently used—the 'open' class. Words from the pivot class almost always appear in combination with words from the open class and never alone or with each other. Words from the open class, however, may appear alone and with each other. . . . Pivot classes may appear first or second in sentences, but no word from a single pivot class appears in both places. The open class is quick to take in new vocabulary while the pivot class is slow to do so." (McNeill, 1970, p. 25)

In short, pivot (P) and open (O) words may be combined: (P+O), (O+P), (O+O). The virtue of this approach is that it represents the first attempt to develop a form of grammar which is based on what the child says rather than using terms derived from adult grammatical analysis. An extensive superstructure of interpretation based on adult thought-forms and concepts subsequently developed, but before this is looked at, it is important to turn to the critics of pivotal grammars.

One of the comments which has been made is that much of the data on pivot grammars is selective, and does not include all the utterances of the children at the two-word stage. Only Braine (1963) himself was discussing a relatively complete list. Bloom (1970) noted a number of discrepancies when she came to look at her data, collected from three children. In addition to the two-word utterances which fitted the pivot-open classification there were others which could not, and these in fact proved to be the majority in two of the children. It was extremely difficult to classify some words; "Mommy" occurred first in 29 out of the 32 earliest examples and was used in other ways characteristic of a pivot word, but there are strong objections to calling it a function word rather than a noun. A third problem relates to the inadequacy of the pivot grammar when two utterances of identical form appear, but with very different meanings or at least, in very different situations. For instance, "Mommy sock" was said when one child, Kathryn, was picking up her mother's sock, and again when her mother was putting Kathryn's sock on for her. In the former the relation which the child was expressing concerned the mother's ownership of the article, a possessive relation; in the other her mother was the agent in doing something with the sock, in grammatical terms expressing the subject-object relation. These two examples show that the same utterance, the "surface structure" of what is said, can derive from very different forms of "deep structure", where the meaning and content of the utterance reside. Bloom found that two-word utterances of the noun-noun type are very common in the early stages and can represent a number of different grammatical relations, the two mentioned being the most common. The de Villiers (1974) also found that in the early stage of two-word utterances 87% of two-word utterances were of the noun-noun type, mostly referring to an animate-subject—inanimate-object type of construction. Children must not only learn the meanings of words, the name or label of a particular object for instance, but they must also learn to convey the meaningful relationships they have observed, and the most appropriate grammatical forms by which these relationships are expressed. It is no wonder that early two-word utterances do not flow thick and fast, but that there is instead a long apprenticeship. As Bloom (1976) says, it is not enough to learn "Mommy". It is also necesarry to learn mother as subject—"Mommy push"; as object—"push Mommy"; as possessor—"Mommy('s)"; as possessed — "my Mommy"; in identity — "Mommy ('s a) lady": and so to express various aspects of "Momminess" in syntactically appropriate ways. The pivot grammar approach is an oversimplification of the way in which children are trying to convey the various relations observed in their environment.

At this stage of language development there is so much ambiguity in children's utterances that it is quite impossible to make out the meaning of what the child is saying purely from the words themselves. The adult listener can interpret and fill in the blanks, but who is to say the interpretation is correct? Bloom overcomes this difficulty by taking careful note of the situation in which an utterance was made. She based her rationale on the oft-repeated observation that children talk about what they are doing and looking at; she concluded that it is generally not difficult to judge the relationship between what a child says, and what he is talking about. "Adults who know children tend to know what they are saying more often than not."

(Bloom, 1970, p. 9)

A sense of caution dictates that those who know children (and to whom can this actually apply in practice?) know the limitations of their knowledge about the well-springs of childhood behaviour and speech. Piaget has made it very clear that the adult interpretation of what a child perceives and understands may be far from the truth: the true developmental approach is astonishingly difficult to acquire, because once any of us have achieved a new cognitive, interpersonal or linguistic skill, we cannot readily dispense with it. If therefore we are to understand the mind of the child on his terms rather than on our own, we may only make the broadest of generalizations about the mapping of our perceptions, thought forms, and verbal constructions on to those of the child and vice versa.

The numerous categories of meaning attributed to the child by those studying their language has been criticized by Howe (1976) as revealing more about the way an adult looks at the child, than about the nature of the child's verbal and cognitive processing abilities. These semantic categories, some of which have been noted above, contain a variety of ambiguities which cannot be resolved by considering the words of the child's utterance alone; not only this but neither can they be resolved by resorting to the situational context in which they are uttered. Does "Shoes Nanny" refer to the locative relation "There are shoes on Nanny" or to the possessive "Nanny has shoes"? In interpreting an utterance like this Bloom would turn back from the actual situation to the word order, and so fall foul of a position in which "although the meanings of the utterances were supposed to be inferred from the antecedent situation, the interpretation of that situation depended on the word order of the utterances" (Howe, 1976). Similar difficulties arise if the adult, from her knowledge of the language, fills out the utterance by expanding it into a reasonable grammatical sentence, and makes the assumption that the situation then referred to by this sentence is the real-life referent of the child's two-word utterance. Howe emphasizes that no attempt to reconstruct the child's utterance from an adult point of view could ever yield the meanings of two-word utterances, because in order to understand the child's speech, there is the ever present demand that one must know how children conceive of reality. It should be noted that the extreme rigour of her approach is directed, not at the parents' intuitive, functional, but relatively loose grasp of what their child is saying, so much as against the attempt to reconstruct that saying precisely in terms of adult language. This is particularly important if a theoretical superstructure is built up on these dubious foundations. Basing her argument on Piaget's descriptions of the emergence of the object concept, and of the young child's grasp of cause and effect (summarized in Chapter 3), she believes that there are only three very general concepts available to the child at the time of the appearance of two-word utterances. Bloom, and Brown (1973), Schlesinger (1971), and Slobin (1970) each list 7 or 8 possible relations. Howe's list of three include "action of concrete object" (regardless of the role of the "object" in the action); "state of concrete object" (whether it be an attribute, a location or a possession); and "name of concrete object". Her restricted list is more in keeping with the child's underlying cognitive abilities, but it needs to be remembered that the child has other uses for language than the conveying of his observations about concrete realtiy.

Teasing, play and the desire to share each other's company must be taken into account in any adequate description of verbal interaction between the child and his mother. The attempts of the serious researcher to unravel the complexities of pragmatics, semantics and syntax overlook the important fact that mother and child are not always very serious when they are talking together—unless perhaps a researcher or clinician is listening to every word. Descriptions of the development of child language are singularly earnest and there is little in the literature to suggest that a great deal of talking is carried on for the sheer pleasure it gives the parents and their child. Play is an essential precursor of language and it is a frequent finding that those children who have difficulty in learning language also show difficulties in understanding the symbolic meaning of the activities, play materials and games which their peers enjoy. Much of language is learned and used in the course of play, whether it be with parents or with other children and the development of the two processes are inseparably linked. Even at the two-word stage children can be adept at using words in a provocative and make-believe way. An example observed whilst sitting in a crowded railway train was that of a girl, less than two years old who looked up at her father in anguish and said "Do wee-wee", then burst into peals of laughter at her father's discomfiture, to the amusement of their fellow passengers. Piaget (1954) quotes a similar example.

The trend in the study of child language has been away from the acquisition of syntax and the ways in which grammars of child language may be written, and towards an understanding of what it is the child is trying to say, and the purposes which underlie his speech acts. This academic trend is to be applauded; the limitations of any approach to language acquisition which single-mindedly ignores other aspects of the child's development as a whole, or the interrelated aspects of language form and function are clearly apparent. Unfortunately, the theoretical insights which have been gained, and they are many, have been remarkably unproductive in the applied sense. Those whose work it is to deal with the day to day problems of assessment and diagnosis, of therapy and teaching have been provided with very little in the way of practical tools which are effective in a qualitative, let alone quantitative way. It should perhaps be said that any theoretical claim which cannot be confirmed in its real-life application to children with disorders of the acquisition and use of language will always remain tentative and unproven. This acid test of a theory is necessary because it is the only way in which it can properly be put on trial, that is, by the child rather than by the theoretician's peers. Nature combines with mankind to make endless experiments in delaying and perturbing language development, and there are innumerable opportunities to try out theory in practice for those who have the courage and humility to do so.

At the present time the most effective approach to assessment and remediation is based on syntactical development. In her consideration of the various options available, Rees (1971) concluded that the most hopeful way to approach the problem was to determine the developmental sequence in which the various syntactic structures appeared and were used by the child. This view is supported by Crystal, Fletcher, and Garman (1976) who go further and say that from the therapist's point of view such an approach is unavoidable. Clearly there is the assumption that the order in which syntactic structures emerge in the speech of the normal child is appropriate also to the child in whom language development is not taking place normally. Instances may occur where this assumption cannot be relied upon, but for the great majority of children it provides an invaluable working rule, and one which is constantly borne out in practice. The aim of Crystal and his colleagues was to develop a procedure for analyzing the syntactic character of language disorders and they chose as their basis a descriptive framework arising out of "the general tradition of structuralist linguistics ... which was the dominant mode of syntactic investigation in the period preceding Chomsky" (Crystal *et al.*, 1976, p. 37). This framework is "A grammar of contemporary English" (Quirk, Greenbaum, Leech, and Svartvik, 1972) which was the culmination of a long-term survey of spoken and written English, intended to function as a reference grammar on normal usage. It is an empirical approach, stating the facts as they are rather than interpreting them on the basis of any particular linguistic theory. Crystal and his co-workers adopt a similar approach in their description of syntactic structures in the child, describing what is said by the child admittedly in terms of adult language, but detailing very clearly the order of emergence of the various ways a child will join words together, and the emergence of the various parts of speech.

Even at this basic grammatical level a child's two-word utterances turn out to be surprisingly diverse. There is a primary division into clauses and phrases, each of which may then be considered in several ways. The fundamental difference between the two is the presence or absence of a verb. "The verb is the most important part of a clause, because it determines most of the patterns which are allowed to appear in the rest of the sentence." (Crystal *et al.*, 1976, p. 44). Clauses are of three main types: statement—"man gone", "dadda running", "that hot", "give teddy", "mummy car", "not run": question—"what that?", "pussy where?"; command—"jump down". Certain difficulties will immediately be apparent. Whilst at times it may be possible to infer a grammatical structure of the form subject-verb, or verb-object this is not always the case; in some of the examples given (all those of the authors themselves) there is no verb. One is then obliged to infer a structure such as subject-object with the verb implicit rather than said as in "that hot" (where "is" is implied) as also in "pussy where?". Syntactic analysis is in consequence tentative at this stage, and it is not possible to circumvent entirely the ambiguities noted earlier in the work of other writers. It will be seen as an advance on the pivot-open grammar however despite these inherent difficulties. The pivot class contains words of very different types; examples from one of Braine's children (Braine, 1963) include—big, pretty, more, my, see, hi, byebye, allgone, it. It is misleading not to differentiate between these words and to imply that adjectives, verbs, nouns and others all function in the same way. Phrases may be readily apparent if they are of the noun phrase type—red shoes; mummy('s) bag; or are prepositional—in box, on table. Confusion may easily arise however over verb phrases such as "want see" or "come out".

The numerous opportunities for confusion which are an inevitable consequence of the child's ability to put no more than two words together, to which must be added the limitations of his conceptual grasp of the world around him, begin to be resolved as the child develops his use of language. With the appearance of three words in an utterance a more clearly defined sentence structure can be recognized by the parents, who can be adept at providing the details of their child's language development provided that the right questions are asked. A three-word utterance may be formed by the joining together of clause and phrase; "see shoes" and "red shoes" combines to create "see red shoes". A single element of clause structure may be expanded by two elements of phrase structure in various ways: "see that teddy", "sit on chair", "let man go". In addition to this process of blending, Crystal, Fletcher, and Garman describe the appearance of new structures both at clause and at phrase level. Clauses may be statement patterns of the type "teddy want biccy", "daddy gone work", "not ball go"; they may be questions—"where my mummy?", "be doggy gone?"; or commands—"put ball down", "let me go", "don't kick me". At phrase level they might include utterances of the type "big red ball", "that big doggy" or introduce the use of auxiliary verbs—"train be going", They do go". The child becomes more proficient at using words as he masters the underlying structures by which they are put together in a sequence. Not only does he join words together more easily, but he also uses words more readily as a whole, utterances flowing one after the other. This is an example of a sequence observed personally, which needs no additional description because the utterances by themselves are sufficient for the reader to visualize the scenario with complete clarity: "daddy not lid . . . lid not there . . . put some milk in . . . and tea . . . cup tea daddy". From this time on a child's mother will spontaneously comment on how easy it is to have a conversation with him; if language has been late in coming this is a development of considerable psychological importance to her.

In addition to these changes in the ways in which words are joined together, the forms of words themselves will be modified by the child. During the period when the child is using three-word utterances, ranging in age from roughly 2 y 0 m to 2 y 6 m, the sounds of words are altered by the addition of endings which carry a special significance. These inflections, which are themselves governed by certain quite specific phonological rules, are used to indicate plurals—an "-s" or "-z" sound; verb participles—"-ing" or "-ed" (which may sound as "d" or "t"); contraction of the auxiliary verb—"I'm", "he's", and so on for possessives, comparisons of "bigger" and "biggest", and the formation of adverbs by the addition of "-ly" at the end of the word.

6 Deficit and Delay in the Development of Spoken Language

As a species, we are more than could be predicted from an anatomical inventory of our constituent parts and the human animal displays an astonishing development of interpersonal, emotional and cognitive functions. These functions, unique though they are in the animal world, are dependent on the efficient and precisely coordinated working of their component parts. They are doubly vulnerable since they are at the mercy of the host of factors which may damage the various systems and organs of the body, and carry their own fragility as the price to be paid for their recent appearance in evolutionary time. They are tempered in the crucible of a few million years of usage at most, a small fragment of the hundreds of millions of years of vertebrate development which undergird vision, digestion and the neuromuscular processes of mobility.

Prevalence of Disorder

Epidemiological studies of the prevalence of language disorder are limited. Morley (1972) published the results of her survey of all children born in the city of Newcastle during the two months of May and June, 1947. When these children were aged 3 y 6 m to 3 y 10 m there were 181 (19.2%) out of a total of 944 who had some form of delay or defect in spoken language. MacKeith and Rutter (1972) reviewed the available data and their necessarily tentative conclusions are summarized in Table 6.1. In order to give an indication of the total number involved for one single year of age, the annual number of live births is assumed to be 900,000 in the United Kingdom.

These figures, though not precise, are sufficient to give an indication of the size of the problem; if anything they are likely to be an underestimate. Furthermore they relate to the prevalence of language disorder and speech difficulties at the time of school entry, which in the United Kingdom is at age five years. The figures quoted above from Morley indicate that the problem is very much larger in children ap-

Table 6.1. *Estimated prevalence of disorders of spoken language in the five year old child derived from MacKeith and Rutter (1972)*

Category of child	Number per 1,000	Total number* at 5 y
1 Attending ordinary school		
a) Speech unintelligible to strangers	40	36,000
b) Severely retarded language	10	9,000
2 Associated with mental retardation	15	13,500
3 deafness	1	900
4 cerebral palsy	1	900
TOTAL	67 (6.7%)	60,300

* Based on 900,000 births p.a. in the United Kingdom.

proaching their fourth birthday. This age is of particular significance because there is so little time remaining to refer, assess and initiate effective forms of treatment before the child is due to start at school. We need to develop an approach to disorders of spoken language which is preventive. Once such a highly overlearned skill has been acquired, and the strategies which the child develops to circumvent his particular difficulties become programmed into the neuropsychological routines subserving speech, then the therapeutic problems are increased by an order of magnitude. It is then not simply (though it rarely is simple) a matter of helping the child to produce suitable forms of spoken language through which he may express himself. It is necessary first to erase the deeply entrenched but faulty patterns of production before correct patterns of production can replace them. This emphasizes the therapeutic difficulties and takes no account of the years of the child's lifetime during which he and his parents and those others around have been quite unable to enjoy a normal communication system. The frustration, bewilderment, annoyance and guilt which this causes can be extreme, and leads to the usually completely erroneous judgment that the child's trouble is emotional in origin. This is to commit the cardinal error of confusing effect and cause.

It is we, not the child, who demonstrate a curious emotional bias to the problems of language acquisition and use. The universal reaction is one of disbelief, expressed in the form that the difficulty is only temporary in nature, and that the child will soon grow out of it. The danger is that this widely held attitude is partially true. Morley's figures show that nearly one in every five children had some problem with spoken language at the age of (on average) 3 y 9 m; using the estimates provided by MacKeith and Rutter this figure had fallen to about 7% by the time of school entry. These proportions refer to very large numbers of individual children. If they related to delay in the acquisition of a more obviously physical skill such as walking they would cause widespread scandal, let alone if they were the estimates of prevalence of some non-lethal but life-limiting disease such as chronic nephritis or tuberculosis of the spine. The attitudes of society at large are reflected in the medical approach to these different conditions. The far-reaching importance of dealing with physical conditions precisely and efficiently is appreciated, and modern health care has achieved a remarkable level of proficiency. Indeed this point in time probably marks the zenith of technical accomplishment in many respects and future gains will be smaller and more costly in terms of money, equipment and manpower. Failure of full, normal development of the uniquely human skills, seen for instance in mental retardation or more specifically for our purpose, in the acquisition of speech, arouses no sense of urgency. On the contrary the characteristic response is that there is no problem and that all will soon be well with the child.

The Nature of Society's Response

Before examining in more detail the manifestations of language delay and disorder it is necessary to pause for a moment to consider the nature of this phenomenon. It is interesting in its own right and is of the greatest consequence to the afflicted child and his parents. The great majority of parents seen in clinical practice encounter grave difficulties in obtaining careful assessment and constructive advice when they voice their fears about their child's poor progress in spoken language. The community as a whole takes it upon itself to reassure the parents that there is nothing wrong, and even if there is, that in three or six months he will be talking just like every other child. The delay is real enough and can be given numerical expression. In the report of a study carried out by medical audiologists of the nine countries of the European Common Market (CEC Report, 1980), 24% of the 2,988 children were suspected, mostly by their parents, of having a hearing loss before the age of one year, and approximately two thirds of the children by their third birthday. Despite the fact that none of the children had a hearing loss of less than 50 dB, that the majority were suffering from congenital sensorineural deafness and were showing severe delay in learning to talk, and that screening programmes are widely used to ensure early detection, less than 50% had had their hearing loss diagnosed by their third birthday. Thereafter, the number remaining to be diagnosed fell by only about 5% each year, so that it was not until the children were 6 years of age that over 90% of them had finally been diagnosed as deaf (see Fig. 6.1).

The attitude is so widespread that it seems likely one has to seek an explanation at an anthropological level, rather than point an accusing finger at doctors, teachers,

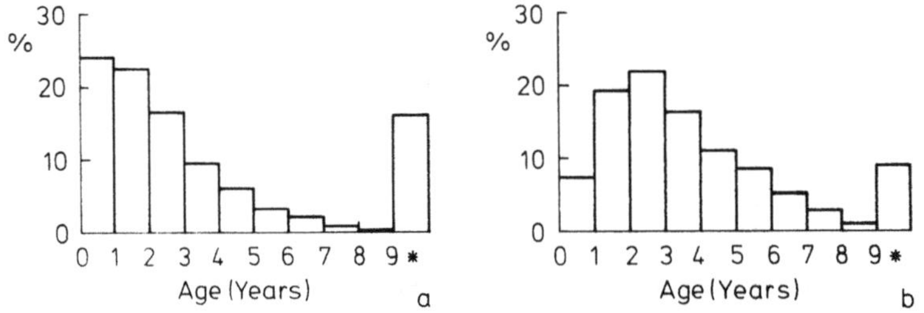

Fig. 6.1. Comparison of age at which hearing loss first suspected and age at which hearing loss confirmed for 2,988 children in the countries of the European Community (CEC). *a* Age loss first suspected, *b* age loss confirmed. (From CEC Report *Childhood Deafness in the European Community 1980)*

therapists or mothers-in-law for their lack of concern. It is as if the belief in the human ability to talk is so deeply rooted, so intrinsic and necessary a part of our make-up, it is inconceivable that a child can fail to acquire speech. There is a regression from rationality to magic, which is never quite so far away as one might hope, and the words of reassurance are the twentieth century equivalent of the incantation which will cure the affliction. To give weight to the cure's effectiveness there is frequently added an instance of the widespread myth of sudden and total resolution demonstrated by some child who did not talk till 5 years (say) and later became famous for his literary or oratorical gifts. One cannot deny the possibility; it may be true. At a personal level, however, I have never yet seen it happen, despite being involved over numerous years with the assessment and follow-up of thousands of children with many different types and degrees of impaired acquisition of language.

The parents are usually the ones to be most concerned, and if they give voice to their concern it is only right that their opinion should be respected for it is they who encounter at first hand every day the evidence of their child's increasing difficulties in learning to talk. We need to be more sensitive to their anxiety, and careful to suppress the primeval instinct which cannot accept the possibility that this uniquely human skill will fail to develop. The child and his parents need the support and guidance of informed professional opinion at least as much as if the condition were some serious physical ailment. The effects of impaired communication are too serious, too far-reaching and long lasting to be treated in any other way.

The Emotional Effect of Impaired Communication

The child cannot give expression to his problems other than through the disturbances of his emotional and communicative behaviour, and it is peculiarly difficult to understand the extent of the disability. Some idea may be conveyed by the experiences of the adult who has difficulty in communicating naturally with his friends and acquaintances through spoken language. The stroke patient, the person who has undergone a laryngectomy, the deaf adult, are examples of different types of disordered interpersonal communication. The effects were poignantly expressed by Ludwig van Beethoven in a letter to his brothers Carl and Johann, written in 1802.

"For the last six years I have been afflicted with an incurable complaint which has been made worse by incompetent doctors ... finally I have been forced to accept the prospect of a permanent infirmity... Though endowed with a passionate and lively temperament and even fond of the distractions offered by society I was soon obliged to seclude myself and live in solitude. If at times I decided just to ignore my infirmity, alas! how cruelly was I then driven back by the intensified sad experience of my poor hearing... Moreover my misfortune pains me doubly inasmuch as it leads to my being misjudged. For me there can be no relaxation in human society, no refined conversations, no mutual confidences. I must live quite alone and may creep into society only as often as sheer necessity demands; I must live like an outcast." (Tyson, 1967)

Beethoven in these words writes for all deaf people, but not only the deaf; the problems of the individual who has any form of difficulty with spoken language are essentially the same. It makes no difference whether the obstacle is to hear and understand what is being said, or to formulate and express one's ideas, observations and desires. We who are able to perform these communicative acts normally, free from any impediment, are immensely intolerant of anything which hinders the easy interchange of speech. It soon becomes reduced to a leaden, lifeless activity shorn of all interest and enjoyment, and embarrassing to speaker and listener alike. The world is so sympathetic to Beethoven (in retrospect) because of his pre-eminence as a creative writer of music. But music was not the main source of his suffering; he could imagine and represent it internally in a way which very few are able to do. It was the lack of understanding, the misjudgements of his fellows which drove him to contemplate suicide. He could find no relaxation in human society but was forced to live alone, as he says; his life was deprived of any communitive activity, any opportunity of the simple pleasure of being with other people, because of the immense barrier raised by the impaired communication. This is the root problem of all in whom the facility for spoken language is impaired or disrupted in some way, and it makes no difference whether the one afflicted is honoured throughout history because of his accomplishments, or is an unknown two-year old struggling to talk.

The Detection of Delay

How does one come to a decision that a particular child is slow in learning to talk? The predominant factor is the concern of the child's parents. If they have voiced the fear that their child is unduly slow their voice should be listened to and some simple screening procedure applied so that a reasonable decision can be reached on whether or not the parent's fears are justified. A few carefully chosen questions are all that are required. How many words can he say? When did he begin to say them? When did he first begin to join two words together spontaneously (as opposed to the saying of simple, learned phrases)? Does he use his voice readily for communication, whether or not actual words are said? Is it easy to understand what he is trying to say? Can he understand what others say to him, even in the absence of gesture and well known domestic or situational cues? Can he hear— not just a plane passing overhead, or the ambulance on its way to an emergency—but quiet sounds and the whispered voice? The answers given to these questions must be in reasonable accordance with the norms of language development, before one is in a position to reassure the parents that all is well. But a child who says no words at 21 months or is not yet joining words at 27 months is decidedly slow, and if he is not able to understand what is said to him his problem is more urgent still.

If we behaved as though the pathology of spoken language was of fundamental significance to a species which relies predominantly upon speech and language, we should be able to come to accurate decisions about the probability of impending delay and disorder not by the second birthday, but in many by the first. At the present time this is clearly a theoretical ideal, but it is not unreasonable to look forward to the time when knowledge of the development and capabilities of these very young children is sufficiently detailed and widespread to make it a practical possibility. The benefits resulting from the introduction of simple guidance principles designed to improve the various features of interpersonal communication, both preverbal and linguistic, whenever the necessity began to be apparent would be far reaching.

The reality is different. Not only are we curiously reluctant to admit the possibility that speech and language are failing to develop at the average, normal rate. The majority of mothers are, at a conceptual level, oblivious to the wealth of sound producing activity which their young children are uttering. This attitude was encountered from the time one first sought to obtain recordings of early vocal activity. The initial response is frequently of the type "I'm afraid you're wasting your time—there will be nothing to record", yet in one of the recordings it is difficult to hear the mother say "He's not saying very much today" because of the flow of inflected, rhythmical babble coming from her child. In the clinic it is rarely worth the effort to obtain any precise description of pre-speech activity, and parents often tend to assume that crying, laughter, shrieks and squeals are the only non-verbal behaviour which merits being reported. This is all the more astonishing because parents are highly sensitive to the vocal activity of their child and respond very readily to it, as has been demonstrated in Chapter 4. Why it should be dismissed so readily, when the first smile, the ability to grasp, to sit up or to take the first step are often charted so precisely must remain a matter for conjecture. It is probably compounded of the lack of any adequately descriptive vocabulary that the parents can use to describe their observations, and the indifference of our culture—that is, of human culture as a whole, whether the child be from Africa or Europe (and for all I know, Asia and the Americas as well)—to any vocal activity which is not truly linguistic. There is a widespread contempt for "baby talk", though virtually all adults and older children modify their speech in a number of more or less appropriate ways when they talk to a little child. It seems possible that once again, our deep-rooted attitudes are casting their superstitious shadows and obscuring the truth of the situation. It is as if the status of language must be preserved at all costs, and its precision may in no way be tampered with, not even by a four-month-old enjoying himself enormously as he produces strings of highly patterned vocal activity, with precisely graded changes of pitch, and accurately timed sequences of sounds. The child must speak properly, or he is not talking at all—except to his parents, wiser and more understanding, in the privacy of their own home.

The "Cause" of Delay and Disorder

Spoken language touches upon so many aspects of human activity that to attempt to label a particular dysfunction or feature as the cause is to oversimplify and distort the clinical reality of the problem. It is frequently asserted that the cause of a child's speech trouble is that he is backward or lazy, or the mother is not stimulating him; the cause may be attributed to sibling rivalry following the birth of another child, or to deprivation, or arise out of the time when his mother was away from home for a week or two. More often than not these "causes" are labels indicating the judgement the clinician has passed on the child and his family, and are far from being an objective and rational assessment of the nature of the condition. Many of the causes which are deemed responsible for a child's impaired language acquisition come into this category, and one needs to beware of them. If one considers such factors as these to be causative, one must be able to explain the mechanisms by which they disrupt the normal processes of language development. They may indeed be causative but unless such assertions really tell us something about the pathogenesis of the child's disability they are of very little value. The gap between cause and effect is too large to be credible.

There is another variant of the "cause" problem which spells difficulty for the medically qualified, and which far from lacking any scientific rigour is in a sense, unjustifiably rigorous. When the physician is faced with a group of symptoms and signs of disease, it is sound practice to avoid attributing a different cause to each component of the overall clinical picture. Instead it should be the aim to try and bring all the different features into relation with one another by looking for a single unifying cause which can explain them all. The same principle applies in the medical approach to the diagnosis of language disorder, but with much reduced strength. This is partly through lack of knowledge, because we are woefully ignorant of for example, which specific neurological processes or microstructures are at fault when we come to consider the fundamental basis of the disorder. This is not to make the mistake of assuming that all disturbances of impaired verbal communication originate at a biomolecular and neurochemical level, but very many more will ultimately come to be explained in this way rather than by loosely asserting some vague, over-generalized "cause".

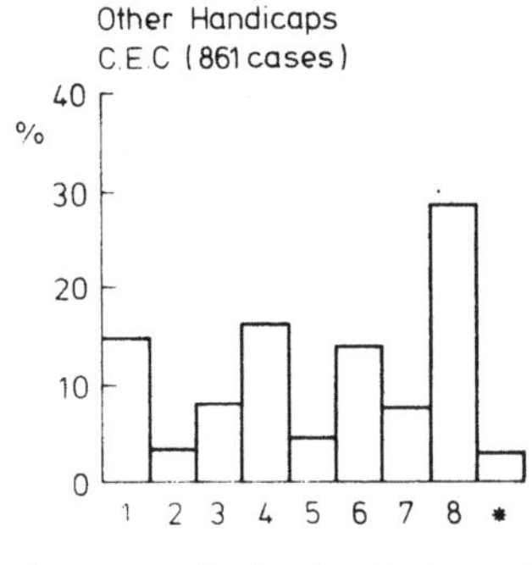

Code for Handicaps

1 Mental only
2 Mental + Visual
3 Mental + Other
4 Visual only
5 Visual + Other
6 Cerebral Dysfunction[a]
7 Behaviour Disorder
8 Others[b]
* Missing data

[a] Cerebral Dysfunction: includes *e.g.* cerebral palsy, hydrocephalus, epilepsy.
[b] Others: includes *e.g.* cardiac, renal, stature, skeletal, skin, gut, blood or language abnormalities.

Deaf children, showing the nature of additional handicaps (CEC Report, 1980)

The three major handicaps (either alone or in combination with others) are:

i) Mental retardation,
ii) Visual deficits,
iii) Cerebral dysfunction (including cerebral palsy, epilepsy, hydrocephalus, etc.).

Fig. 6.2. Distribution of additional disabilities in 861 out of 2,988 children with hearing loss. (From CEC Report *Childhood Deafness in the European Community 1980*)

Apart from our lack of detailed knowledge of the precise mechanisms involved, there is another consideration which limits the value of the "single pathology" approach. There may be not one, but a group of disabilities, and this is such a common finding that one needs actively to acknowledge the fact and conscientiously examine or assess the child as a whole. He may be deaf, but there may also be some degree of visual impairment, or of intellectual function, or he may be mildly spastic. There may be renal dysfunction, abnormalities of skeletal structure, or epilepsy. In the European Common Market study of the children with hearing loss already referred to (CEC Report, 1980), there were no less than 861 children reported as having a handicap additional to deafness. This figure represents 29% of the total number of children. The details are shown in Fig. 6.2.

The Antecedents of Disorder

Some of the confusion which clouds discussion and which may already have become apparent to the reader is semantic. What is meant precisely by such words as "the diagnosis" and "the cause"? May one speak in the same breath of some abnormality of neurotransmitter formation and release at nerve synapses along the neuromotor pathway, and of some emotional disturbance affecting the behaviour of the child as a whole, and call them both "cause"? These are dysfunctions operating at very different levels of human organization. It would appear to be highly desirable and logically proper not to use the same verbal concept to label such very different processes, the one molecular, the other at the level of the psyche. The use of the word "cause" cannot be avoided altogether because it is the question which parents will inevitably and rightfully ask. But until we know and understand the causal mechanisms whether the lesion be at the neurochemical level or at the psychosocial level of interaction between child and parent, meaningful discussion is best centred on the *antecedents* of the disorder. The antecedents are all the relevant contributory factors, operating together, which can in the present state of our knowledge provide a reasonable explanation of this one individual and particular child's impaired acquisition and use of spoken language.

In the following pages an approach to diagnosis and assessment is considered, not because of its value in clinical practice (this is not the purpose of our study), but because of the insights it may provide on the nature and antecedents of the child's disability. It has been developed empirically over the years in response to the problems encountered, in order to arrive at a better understanding of the processes which disturb the normal acquisition of language. It is useful also in coming to decisions on the regime of treatment, therapy and education which will enable the child to achieve a higher level of performance in linguistic and communication skills, though it would be turning too far aside from our theme to consider these aspects further. It must suffice to state an acid test of the significance of any theoretical systems model in medicine. If the model proves to have no practical value in the amelioration of disease or disability it is either inaccurate or too speculative and fails to represent the clinical components and their inter-relationships sufficiently closely.

The Nature of Developmental Delay

At this point it is necessary to digress briefly and consider what is meant by developmental delay. In charting the maturation and development of a child it is helpful to have some yardstick by which parents, doctors and others may assess his progress. This is not represented by a figure for average age derived from looking at large numbers of children, but is best thought of as a range such as that used by Touwen (1976) in which the age is given when 80% of children achieved a particular, defined activity. There are a number of variations on this theme, so that one may determine the age at which first 50% and then all of the sample population of normal children have achieved a particular landmark. Developmental norms properly used are the equivalent in other branches of medicine of the normal range of values in the cellular or chemical constituents of the blood, cerebrospinal fluid or other body fluids and tissues and indicate the extent of deviation from the norm. When a child fails to achieve a particular norm, it does not mean that a specifically "developmental" process is at work; the one does not follow from the other. There are a number of pathological processes which result in a child falling behind in reaching a certain milestone such as walking; he may have had congenital dislocation of the hip or be spastic, or to give an even more gross example he may be a thalidomide child, and simply not have legs. Though these conditions have marked developmental effects, they are not developmental disorders. There is a widespread but largely unrecognized tendency to use the adjective "developmental" in the same way as "idiopathic", the difference being that in the latter case the unknown nature of the underlying condition or process is frankly acknowledged in the meaning of the word. To describes a child as having a "specific developmental expressive disorder" is spuriously precise and says nothing about the underlying nature of the disordered language function, other than that the child is slow in learning to talk. The danger of such terminology lies in the assumption that the condition is sufficiently defined at a conceptual level and no thought is given to underlying mechanisms, whether these be cognitive or neurological. There can be no doubt that in the course of time the precise pathogenesis of many of these conditions will be elucidated, and our terminology, such as it is, will be shown up as grossly overgeneralized. At the present time we would probably best describe the child's language disability by relating it to a number of functions, and from these to elaborate a series of syndromes which could provide a practical, state-of-the-art but incomplete description of the child's condition (Martin, 1980).

The Pattern and Extent of the Disability

The Child's Speech and Language

Since the primary concern of the parents, or the health clinic doctor, health visitor, therapist or nursery teacher, is the child's slowness in learning to talk, it is appropriate to start by assessing his spoken language. One should endeavour to gain an accurate description of the child's speech from his parents. This would appear to be a simple enough task. One needs reasonably precise information on the size of his vocabulary, but the first difficulty is immediately encountered. It may appear that he is able to say a large number of words; it is important to distinguish between those words the child imitates in response to his mother, and those which he says spontaneously and uses meaningfully. That a child is able to imitate words clearly and readily gives valuable information about speech perception and the functioning of the neuromuscular pathways to the speech apparatus, but it says nothing about the child's linguistic performance. The sound pattern he has reproduced is not a word until it encapsulates some element ofmeaning. And so it is for all utterances which the child may make, even if they are several words long, just as the family parrot calls out "Do you want a cup of coffee?" or "Can I have the car?". His subsequent behaviour has failed so far to reveal any great interest in either. Dating the time when the first words began to be used poses similar problems because of the confusion with babbling on the one hand and the occurrence of imitation on the other. Difficulty arises in another way over children who have severe difficulties in the physical production of words; a mother may be extremely reluctant to report that her child is saying words because they are poorly formed and she is the only one who can understand what he is saying. Defective articulation creates even greater difficulties when it comes to trying to assess the number of words a child is putting together. It may be possible for him to say individual words recognizably, but as words are joined into two- and three-word utterances and longer, the intelligibility may drop sharply. Under these circumstances the speech therapist has the greatest difficulty on deciding on the level of the child's syntactical development and his grasp of linguistic structures; all but the most salient words are unrecognizable so that prepositions and auxiliary verbs cannot be detected, nor can the presence of appropriate word endings, such as verb inflections or the construction of plurals.

Assessment

If there is to be any accuracy of assessment it is necessary not only to obtain an accurate history from the parents but also to obtain objective evidence of the child's spoken language directly from him. When we listen to a young child our attention is directed to what it is the child is saying and, usually quite unconsciously, we abstract the meaning of his speech. In reporting that speech, the tendency is invariably to clothe the child's utterance in the correct grammatical form as the listening adult has understood, not as she has heard it. The trained listener, and it requires a good deal of experience with children to achieve this capability with adequate precision, has to listen to no less than five levels of spoken language at the same time, as it were. There is the prime necessity to abstract the semantic content, what meaning it is that the child is trying to convey. Then there are the actual words, the way they are ordered or arranged in the utterance, whether they are nouns, verbs, determiners, adjectives and their functional significance as agent, action and so on. There is the structure of the word itself and the accuracy of its formation in such words as "gived" or "see(e)d" or "sockses". At this level there is also the occurrence of infantilisms so-called, such as "shoe-shoe" for shoe or "lummerly" for lovely. These merge into the early difficulties associated with articulation such as "weez" for "squeeze me", "habit" for "have it" or "didi dese?" for "what are these?". The precision of articulation needs to be assessed, the manner of formation of particular types of segmental sound, such as plosives and fricatives, continuants, and vowels, those which are omitted or substituted, and the regularity or haphazard nature of errors. The final level, no less important but one which is frequently overlooked in an unduly segmental approach to the analysis of speech, is the prosodic features of fluency and rhythm, syllabic patterning and stress, intonation and volume, laryngeal tone and nasality, in association with respiratory capacity and control of breath.

The Approach to the Child

Talking is not merely a matter of the words uttered and their intelligibility, but the way in which the child shows his willingness to cooperate and to enter into a relationship, to play with the various play materials made available to him, and to communicate verbally. This is a crucial issue: we have tended to assume that the child, brought by his parents to the outpatient clinic, will talk in these unfamiliar surroundings to unfamiliar adults. It is characteristic of the child who has any difficulty with speech that he will demonstrate awareness of his difficulty by remaining silent, or reluctantly resorting to one-word utterances. The slightest evidence the child detects of being put under pressure, of being made to talk, is sufficient to reduce him to uncompromising silence forthwith. One is completely at the mercy of the child, and it is essential to respect his difficulties and to allow time for a mutual relationship to develop so that he can give of his best. The difference between theory and practice is never more clearly seen that in the way one clinician can help to resolve the child's anxieties, and have him cooperating actively and talking readily without her appearing to make any effort at all, whilst another is faced by a tight-lipped, moist-eyed child who seeks the reassurance of his mother's lap. The fundamental difference in approach is probably that between invitation and coercion, and the child soon becomes aware of this.

It is not intended to consider in any depth the practical aspects of clinical assessment; they are fascinating but outside the aim of our discussion. The brief description given will indicate the nature of the information required and the reality of the problems associated with an accurate delineation of the child's spoken language. The principles contained therein apply with equal force to the various other aspects of the child's behaviour and cognitive performance which need to be assessed.

The Child's Understanding of Speech

In the first approximation to a working model of the child's disability, the other component, apart from verbal expression, which must be examined and evaluated is his ability to understand what is said to him. Parents tend, almost without exception, to overestimate a child's verbal comprehension and will give examples (it is essential to obtain specific examples of the sort of comment or request a mother says her child understands) which may suggest there has been no need for a single word to be said in order to get her child to do what she wanted. The context of the activity, the time of day, the sequence of preceding events, the immediate objects around, what she herself is doing, her facial expression, the gestures of her head, eyes and hands, all combine to give the child a clear indication of what is required of him, even though he is profoundly deaf and cannot hear a word of what she says. Another difficulty lies in the fact that a child may hear and understand, but will be able to respond only to the simplest request of the "go and get. . . .your teddy, your shoes etc." variety when he is at an age that he should be able to carry out very much more complex requests *e.g.* "Go upstairs to mummy's bedroom and bring me the blanket under the bed". It is as necessary to gain an accurate indication of the child's ability to understand what is said to him, and to relate this information to the developmental norms as for his spoken language. A procedure widely used in formal assessment is the Reynell Developmental Language Scale (Reynell, 1969). With these two components of language usage adequately sketched out it is possible to study the relationship between them. It may take several forms: for clinical purposes the algebraic expressions of inequality are simple but effective and revealing, considered in relation to the child's chronological age (CA).

If the child's ability to understand what is said to him is labelled VC (verbal comprehension), and his ability to speak VX (verbal expression), one may formulate his performance—

$$\text{CA} \quad (\text{r}) \quad \text{VC} \quad (\text{r}) \quad \text{VX} \qquad (1)$$

where (r) stands for the relationship between the terms. This relationship may take the following forms—

$=$ the usual sign for equality; meaning that there is no difference in developmental age between the terms. For practical purposes, this may be taken to be within 20% of the age.

$\geqq$ greater than or equal to; meaning that there is some uncertainty about the precise relationship or that it is on the borderline with the next category of impairment.

$>$ greater than; meaning that there is a discrepancy of 20—25% or more between the respective developmental ages and CA.

$\gg$ much greater than; meaning that there is a discrepancy of 40—50% or more.

Some examples will make their use clearer.

$$\text{CA} = \text{VC} > \text{VX} \qquad (2)$$

The child is able to understand in an age-appropriate way what is said to him but there is a moderate degree of impairment of his ability to speak. If CA is 3 y 0 m, it may be that his level of spoken language is equivalent to that of a normal child of 2 y 3 m.

$$\text{CA} > \text{VC} = \text{VX} \qquad (3)$$

This represents a child in whom the ability to understand is impaired, by perhaps 25% of his CA or rather more, and there is no difference between his ability to understand and to talk.

$$CA > VC > VX \tag{4}$$

The child has a moderate impairment of verbal comprehension, and his ability to talk is further impaired in relation to his level of understanding. Reading from left to right the effect is additive for each relation signified, so that in this example the relation between CA and VX is: CA $\gg$ VX showing that there is severe impairment of verbal expression.

In the formal expression of language disorder in this way, it is necessary to arrange the terms in the order stated, and the other sign of inequality *i.e.* $<$ (less than), is not permitted. It is of course possible for a child to have a language ability well in excess of his actual age, just as one sees children with intelligence quotients of 125 and more. We are here concerned with impairment of ability and the clinical problems associated with it, rather than with the gifted child. It may be argued that it is necessary to represent certain children in such a way that the "less than" sign be used. An example might be

$$CA \gg VC < VX \tag{5}$$

More precise assessment almost invariably reveals that this is either an error of observation, and the child is not really using language in the way that he appears to be speaking it, or it is an artefact (which amounts to the same thing), and the child has been trained by his parents, teacher or therapist to use forms of words which are learned as such rather than being constructed spontaneously from the basic building bricks of his vocabulary, fixed together then and there with the mortar of syntax.

Consideration of a consecutive and unselected series of 315 children, seen in a period of 2½ years and who presented with difficulty in the learning or use of spoken language (partially reported elsewhere, Martin, 1980), revealed that the impairment of their abilities in verbal comprehension and expression was as shown in Table 6.2.

Table 6.2. *Overall distribution of impairment of verbal comprehension and expression in 315 children*

Level of ability	Verbal Comprehension	Verbal Expression
Normal (N)	108	54
Moderate impairment (M)	60	58
Severe impairment (S)	147	203
Total	315	315

The way in which these abilities relate to one another in the individual children is shown in Table 6.3.

Table 6.3. *Distribution of individual profiles of impairment of verbal comprehension and expression*

Verbal Comprehension	Verbal Expression Normal	Moderate	Severe
Normal	54	26	28
Moderate impairment		30	30
Severe impairment		2	145

Method of Scaling Disability

The grading of a particular feature such as verbal expression, or the various components to be considered later, was determined in a number of stages. The information from the clinical history, assessment and examinations was scored on a selected group of items, the actual number of which varies for the different functions or components. The total was adjusted to take account of the different number of data entry points so that comparison is facilitated between the components, and a ten point formal scale is used for this, running from 0—9. Normal ability is represented by 0, and severe impairment by 9. Such a scale is over-precise in practice, and it is more realistic clinically to use the three point scale —"Normal" (*i.e.* within normal limits), "Moderate impairment" and "Severe impairment"—referred to already. The significance of these terms is defined more precisely in Table 6.4.

Table 6.4. *Numerical and verbal grading of impairment*

Developmental quotient, per cent	100		90		80		70		60		50
Formal scale	0	1	2	3	4	5	6	7	8	9	
Clinical scale	Normal ability				Moderate impairment				Severe impairment		

1. "Developmental quotient" refers to the child's level of ability as assessed divided by the chronological age, and multiplied by 100 to express it as a percentage.
2. Hearing loss is entered by using the middle line of the scale to represent the mean loss, in 10 dB steps: it cannot be expressed in developmental or percentage terms.

It is never an easy matter to decide where to place the boundary lines in a magnitude scale of disability, and individuals will differ considerably over the use of verbal labels which translate the numerical value into words. Practical considerations weigh heavily. It is considered that a child who is functioning at 75% of his chronological age has at least a moderate impairment of language development, whilst one who is functioning at the 50% level indubitably has a severe disability.

Once the relations of the CA (r) VC (r) VX formulation have been evaluated, it quickly becomes apparent that there are as many questions remaining, if not more, than have already been answered. But the formulation has not been a waste of time. On the contrary, it has become possible to look more precisely at the probable nature of the child's language disability, and to decide on the ways in which the time clinically available (always less than one would wish) is used most profitably to achieve an accurate delineation of the problem. It is also of particular assistance in helping the parents and others involved with the child to understand the nature of his difficulty, and provides a basis for explanation.

The Antecedents of Disorder Reception and Comprehension 7

In order to arrive at a sufficiently precise definition of the child's disability it is necessary to look more closely at verbal comprehension and expression. Each of the terms VC and VX is not an entity in its own right but represents the aggregate of a number of separate features. The sum total of the constituent features, known or as yet unidentified, is indicated by the developmental level attained by the child in understanding of language, and in his ability to express himself verbally. These two major aspects of the child's language performance may be subdivided into three components or functions. There is the level of sensory and motor functions, and there are the cognitive and communicative functions. These are represented schematically in Fig.7.1.

It is convenient for descriptive purposes to consider in this way the problems associated with the acquisition of spoken language in the child; it is also meaningful in practice and has in fact evolved out of the necessity of creating some semblance of order in a bewildering and complex field of clinical medicine. But like all descriptions it is essentially a summary and can in no way be complete. The conceptual basis for the diagram is the identification of the most conspicuous or significant findings encountered in children who have presented with some form of delay or difficulty in learning to talk, and the resulting schema is inevitably a personal statement. With these limitations in mind, we can resume at the next deeper level

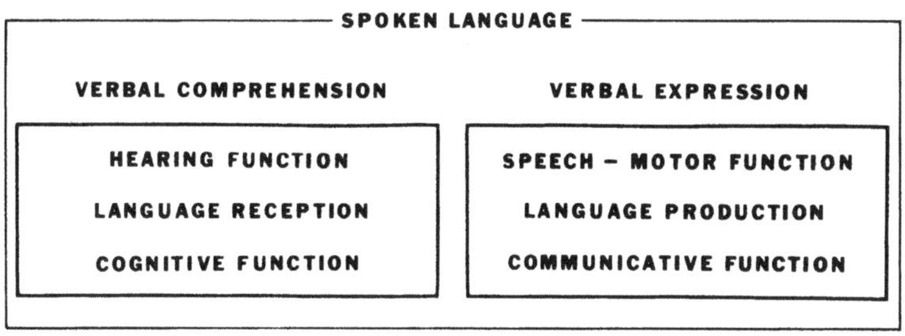

Fig. 7.1. The components or functions of spoken language

the study of language delay and disorder through dysfunction of the various components which are a prerequisite for normal language development. Each of these components has been examined in earlier chapters, and the consideration of certain clinical aspects in the pages which follow relies upon this foundation.

Hearing

For the child who has not yet acquired language deafness is a doubly severe handicap. Being unable to hear all the sounds of the natural and man-made environment he is deprived of a vast input of sensory information which tells him about the nature and activity of the world around him. It is difficult to avoid the conclusion that this restriction of sensory input must have neuro-psychological sequelae which have as yet attracted very little interest or attention. The other consequence is its effect on the learning of language.

The position may be examined in general outline by reference to the series of 315 children mentioned above. Table 7.1 shows the relation of degree of hearing loss on the child's ability to understand what is said to him, and his own ability to talk. In order to avoid the complications of dealing with multiple pathology the children with any measurable degree of intellectual impairment have been excluded.

Table 7.1. *Verbal comprehension and expression in normally hearing and hearing impaired children, with normal intelligence*

Hearing	a) Verbal Comprehension			b) Verbal Expression			Totals for each table (a) and (b)
	Normal	Mod.	Sev.	Normal	Mod.	Sev.	
Normal	76	23	8	29	36	42	107
Moderate (40—75 dB)	22	11	21	18	12	24	54
Severe (80+ dB)	7	2	47	6	2	48	56
Totals	103	36	76	53	50	114	217

The problems of oversimplification and nomenclature are apparent in that there is no recognition of a slight but significant degree of hearing loss at the 20 to 35 dB level. This will account for some of the 23 children with moderate impairment of verbal comprehension. The same problem appears in the children labelled as having a moderate degree of hearing loss. The range of mean auditory threshold is from 40—75 dB, which straddles the level at which the conversational voice is normally used. Some of these children will therefore be able to hear a great deal of what is said to them and around them, whilst at the upper end of the moderately impaired range they may only be able to hear occasional pulses of louder than average speech sound which contributes virtually nothing to the intelligibility of what is being said. It is a fact of clinical experience that some children with hearing losses of 40—45 dB may have severe impairment of verbal comprehension and this is confirmed by the table. There can be no doubt that deafness is an important cause of language disorder, and it is artificial and divisive to separate it off as if it were a separate speciality. Deafness disables language acquisistion primarily because of the sensory deficit it produces. Its effects on language processing and learning, on speech, on aspects of cognitive function, on communication, interaction and emotional development may be similar in particular respects and certain children to other types of language disorder. There has been an undue emphasis on the child's hearing loss and hence on "audiology" at the expense of these other vital aspects.

The Nature of the Handicap

The problems of the deaf child centre round his often severe, and sometimes profound difficulties in learning language. He is in a completely different category from the deafened adult, who may have severe problems in communication and all that this entails, but who is adept in his use of language having mastered its basic rules and functions.

The extent of the deaf child's problems may be more readily appreciated by referring once more to the study of deaf 8 year-old children in the European Community. Table 7.2 has been prepared from the data to indicate the effect which hearing loss has on the child's ability to hear and to understand speech. Though children with hearing losses from 50 dB upward were included in the survey, 75% of them were unable to understand spoken language, other than the 12% who could carry out simple requests. The results for the children when they are wearing their aids shows a definite improvement, and the number who show no evidence of hearing falls from 37% to 10%. Despite this there remain marginally over half the children who at their best have achieved a verbal comprehension level appropriate to a child of 2–3 years old.

Table 7.2. *Hearing capacity of 2988 children aged 8 years, with mean hearing loss of 50 dB or worse in the better ear (CEC Report, 1980)*

Hearing capacity	a) Without hearing aid		b) With hearing aid(s)	
No evidence of hearing	1119	(37.4%)	305	(10.2%)
Hears loud shout at 3 metres	784	(26.2%)	684	(22.9%)
Understands simple requests at 1 metre	358	(12.0%)	635	(21.3%)
Total	2261	(75.7%)	1624	(54.4%)

Examination of the efficacy of hearing aids affords a valuable insight into our inadequate conceptual approach to the effects of sensory deficit. It could be said that the hearing aid has produced problems in the very area it was designed to solve them, and its widespread use has obscured the fundamental issue. This might be formulated in the following way: Given a hearing loss, can the child hear sufficiently well to permit him to perceive and understand speech, to acquire a vocabulary, and to learn the rules governing normal linguistic usage and interpersonal verbal communication? It is necessary to be clear about the meaning of the first part of the question, because on it hangs the rest.

Beyond a certain level of hearing loss it is quite impossible for a child to learn language through listening to the spoken voice. This is an inescapable consequence of the physics of the situation. If the stimulus (*i.e.* the speech signal) is too weak to activate the receiver system (*i.e.* the end-organ located in the inner ear) there is no possibility of onward transmission of the signal, let alone of any form of processing of the signal. Conversation normally takes place at about 55 dB SPL. This level refers to the high energy content sections of the speech signal, associated mostly with the vowels and some of the voiced sounds. Some consonants are very much quieter so that the child never listens to a signal of uniform loudness, but one in which there is an intrinsic variation of 30 dB, quite apart from the modulation of loudness purposefully or unconsciously introduced by the speaker. The vowels carry important information relating to the identification of consonants, particularly in the transitions affecting the second and third formants between the articulation of the consonant (if in initial position) and the steady state achieved during the greater part of the vowel. If the child were only able to hear vowels he would be deprived of vitally important acoustical information; as it is, we cannot assume that hearing is necessarily adequate even for the reception and processing of sounds in the middle and lower regions of the speech frequency range, and of relatively long duration. It can be seen that moderate losses, of the order of 40—50 dB HL may seriously affect the child's ability to learn to talk. The danger of the hearing aid lies in the easy assumption that once it is in position, the child will be able to hear sufficiently well so that the normal processes of speech perception can come into play or if not, that lip-reading will provide the necessary additional information to make good any remaining deficit. This is to overlook, or perhaps never to recognize in the first place, two major obstacles, the one developmental and the other pathological.

The child who has heard nothing of the spoken voice for the first year, or possible two or three years of his life, has been deprived of that amount of listening experience during the time that normally hearing children are showing an astonishing ability to monitor, process and reproduce the basic features of speech, as seen in Chapter 4. In order to do this effectively and consistently, he has to be given innumerable opportunities to listen in the sound forest in which he is located and has to discover how to direct his attention selectively to what is significant for him. By the end of the first year he has learned to model his voice on those around him, to gain control of important features of the speech carrier wave with subtle gradations of pitch, volume, rhythm and voice quality. By the end of the next year he has acquired a sizeable vocabulary, some basic rules of syntax and has learned the rules of joint verbal activity which govern listening and talking, and how to identify the verbal, vocal and non-linguistic cues which indicate the processes of role reversal. He has been practising these skills at a pre-verbal level since well before his first birthday.

The other obstacle is erected by the pathological process which has damaged the sensory end organ or its afferent nerve supply to the brain stem and along the neural pathways within the brain. Some children are able to achieve a remarkably high level of gain with their hearing aids, and despite a severe or even profound loss, manage to learn language at an age appropriate level, and to speak it with no more than the slightest of defects, or none at all (see Table 7.1). Others, often with a hearing loss which as portrayed on the audiogram chart appears to be less severe, never seem to learn to use their aided hearing, appear to have a limited, inadequate level of gain, and have minimal perception of speech. The poor development of language is usually attributed to late diagnosis, inadequate parental care, the wrong hearing aid and failing all this, the co-occurrence of a specific language disorder—as if the child does not already have a highly specific cause for his defective language acquisition. Though the loss of hearing is the conspicuous feature it would be biologically naive to assume that feeding a sufficiently powerful signal into the inner ear will restore the function of the auditory pathways to normal. Such a view takes no account of the disordered endocochlear and neuronal processing which might well accompany the raised threshold for sound. In many children there is a high level of probability that the auditory pathways are not able to filter, extract, reshape and compare (or whatever it is in precise neurophysiological terms this complex collection of nerve tracts and nuclear aggregates of various types of neurones actually does) the appropriate features from the signals fed in by the deranged activity of the sensory cells and nerve fibres in the cochlea.

It is not only the more severe types of sensorineural deafness which affect the child's learning of language. Many children acquire middle ear deafness in infancy, and it is cause for concern to see how many children have evidence of active secretory otitis media during the first year of life. Such children often appear to be poor listeners, inattentive, slow and unresponsive to sound, and show delay in learning to talk, particularly if the condition is more than usually persistent or recurrent.

Hearing Disorder in the Absence of Loss

If we turn away from the child with a clearly demonstrable degree of "deafness" (the term is usually considered synonymous with hearing loss) and look at the children presenting with impairment of verbal comprehension, it will be found that there are a number in whom the auditory threshold and the performance IQ are well within normal limits. In some of these children the hearing dysfunction is so severe that not only are they unable to understand what is said to them, but sounds themselves appear to convey little information. Such children comprise the group variously labelled receptive aphasia or receptive language disorder, congenital auditory imperception and word-deafness (Worster-Drought and Allen, 1929). It is without doubt a rare condition; personal experience reveals that in the majority the diagnosis is incorrect and the true cause is severe peripheral deafness. In the few children in whom there is no hearing loss worse than 20—25 dB, a number of characteristic features are to be found. It can be difficult to separate those with failure of verbal comprehension from autistic children. This is not altogether surprising since amongst the deficits which typify childhood autism, lack of response to sound and severe impairment of language development are prominent. Bartak, Rutter, and Cox (1975) have compared the characteristics of the two conditions in a careful study of 19 autistic (mean age 7 y 0 m) and 23 receptive "dysphasic" children (mean age 8 y 2 m) selected for normal intelligence. Both groups showed a severe and persisting language disorder; the "dysphasic" children were much less behaviourally disturbed, more (relatively) mature and responsive; the autistic children showed gross social and behavioural abnormalities, with rigid and severe ritualistic and compulsive activities; the quality of language, when it developed, was markedly different in that the autistic group showed a more extensive abnormality of language usage with echolalia, reversal of personal pronouns (*e.g.* saying "you" instead of "I") and inappropriate remarks; an inability to speak spontaneously to others, particularly in any responsive, interactive way; and greater difficulty in talking about personal events which had taken place elsewhere or at a different time.

Ricks (1972, 1979) in his study of normal infants and young autistic children showed that though the latter were unresponsive to their parents' voices, this could not be attributed to failure to process sound. On the contrary, they were able to recognize and imitate quite accurately their own apparently meaningless patterns of vocalization, when they heard them on play-back from tape recordings. He considers that they are capable of refined acoustic recognition. This conclusion tends to support Rees in her view that there is no adequate evidence for any auditory factor underlying language disorder:

"The search for a single auditory skill, or even a set of auditory abilities, that is essential to language learning, or impaired in all or most language-disordered children seems futile." (Rees, 1973)

She is clearly not including the deaf child. There is an overly speculative view which attributes a variety of problems in phonology and the production of speech to errors and deficits in auditory perception, even when the child is able to identify spoken words accurately as in speech audiometry and there is no impairment of verbal recognition. Her argument is in part directed against this position, but it would be wrong to assume that because there is no peripheral hearing loss, the remainder of the immensely complicated neural pathways subserving audition, from the cochlear nuclei in the brain stem to the primary auditory cortex on the upper surface of the temporal lobe, must be working normally. Problems in the control of auditory attention, of the ability to recognize and discriminate between sounds, or to retain more than the shortest verbal utterances containing perhaps only two key words, of the difficulties children show in the correct reproduction of sequential patterns of sound (let alone words) all provide circumstantial evidence that some aspects of auditory processing may be impaired. The argument that all these difficulties are caused by disorder at the linguistic level of syntax resolution and extraction of meaning begs too many questions. In the light of observations of those experienced therapists and teachers who are well versed in the problems of children with receptive language disorder, the possibility of auditory dysfunction is real enough.

Griffiths (1972) considers that:

"For at least some aphasic children the focal point of dysfunction may be highly specific, possibly lying in the acoustic encoding of temporal patterns rather than in any fundamental disorder of auditory perception of linguistic capacity as such."

Present day routine clinical tests of hearing give essential information on the threshold of sensation; speech audiometry as it is most widely used and interpreted originates from the same conceptual basis. There is no non-verbal audiological procedure which allows the investigation of hearing function in its discriminatory or perceptual aspects, in those patients in whom the possibility of disorder arises. This is not a problem which is restricted to children, but is almost certainly relevant to certain types of adult aphasic, and may be a hidden factor in many deaf people, the hearing loss obscuring an additional auditory processing problem. Martin and Martin (1973) were in consequence led to explore the possibility of assessing aspects of auditory perception in normally speaking young people. A number of discrimination tasks were constructed involving the response "same", or "different", to pairs of sounds. The three tasks used in the investigation included the ability to detect differences of pitch of a complex sound, temporal duration and rhythmic pattern. To take the first, the basic features of a synthesized, steady-state vowel-like sound were held constant with the exception of the fundamental frequency. The second member of the pair of sounds might differ from the first by 1 Hz, 2 Hz, 4 Hz or 10 Hz, or remain the same. The tests were administered to a group of 14 boys with a mean age of 16.2 y (range 15—18 y). The results revealed a wide range of ability between subjects in the performance of any one type of discriminatory task although the group was essentially uniform with respect to intellectual ability and linguistic development. Perhaps more surprisingly several subjects showed a wide variation in ability in their individual performance of the three different tasks.

Tallal and Piercy (1973, 1974, 1975) have specifically investigated auditory perception in a group of developmental dysphasic children. It is not possible to gain a clear picture of the clinical profiles of the children and they should probably not be regarded as a homogenous group, but this does not invalidate the importance of their findings. These have recently been summarized in Tallal and Piercy (1978). The investigations were based on the hypothesis that the children were defective in the temporal processing of speech, and a number of experiments were carried out to determine more precisely the nature of the deficit. The dysphasic children were found to perform as well as matched controls in their discrimination of two synthesized, steady-state vowels each lasting 250 ms, whatever the duration of the silent interval between the two. If a consonant lasting 40 msec (either "b" or "d") was placed before a vowel (which remained the same throughout this particular test), the dysphasic children performed significantly worse. There are two possible reasons for this: either the duration of the initial segment is too short, or the children are unable to process the continuously changing types of sound characterized here by formant transition between the voiced initial consonant until the formants achieve a steady-state in the remainder of the vowel. This was investigated by replacing the consonant with a brief vowel segment producing in effect a diphthong, and ensuring the initial 40 msec vowel segment changed abruptly from its steady-state to that of the sustained, second vowel without any transition. Once again the task difference was situated in the first 40 msec, and the dysphasic children performed badly. Returning to the consonant-vowel stimuli, if the duration of the initial "b" or "d" was increased from 40 msec to 80 msec there was no significant difference in ability between the dysphasic children and the control group. Their conclusion was that the results "are most easily understood as a failure to make perceptual use of acoustic information which is very brief in duration and rapidly changing" (Tallal and Piercy, 1978, p. 75).

Impaired Auditory Processing and Speech Perception

Children in whom there is some defect in the perception of individual segments of words would almost certainly have (and for practical purposes should be assumed to have) difficulty in the comprehension of spoken language. In the series of 315 children they would therefore be found within the group in whom verbal comprehension is impaired. If, for simplicity's sake, we consider only those with normal intelligence and no loss of hearing there remain 107 children, Table 7.3. Of them, there are 13+10+8 children (31 or 29%) in whom the possibility of an auditory processing problem arises. All of these would necessarily have a distorted phonological system or "speech defect". By sorting the 31 children into those who have or do not have an apparent articulatory problem it should be possible to identify a group within which there is the likelihood of an auditory processing deficit. There were 11 children with no evidence of a speech-motor defect, leaving 20 (18.7%) of whom some, but not necessarily all, could have a disorder of speech perception. There are without doubt others amongst the mentally handicapped, and amongst the deaf.

Table 7.3. *The relation of verbal expression to verbal comprehension in the 107 out of 315 children with normal intelligence and hearing*

	Verbal Expression		
Verbal Comprehension	Normal	Mod. imp.	Severe imp.
Normal	29	23	24
Moderately impaired		13	10
Severely impaired			8

Sequential, Auditory Memory

There is another aspect of temporal processing, which might be described as being at the macroscopic rather than the microscopic level of very brief durations in the production of plosive consonants. This relates to the problem of serial memory performance. Using the task in which the dysphasic children performed well, *i.e.* for steady-state vowels, Tallal and Piercy produced sequences with various combinations of the two vowel sounds. Three, four or five of these elements were contained in a sequence, which was then compared with another vowel combination of the same length. The dysphasic children had no difficulty with the three and four element sequences, but their performance was impaired for the sequences with five elements. This could be attributed to two possible reasons: either the children have a memory problem when the sequence exceeds a certain length, or they need a disproportionately longer time to process the longer sequences. In their investigation of these possibilities, Tallal and Piercy found some evidence to support the hypothesis that the dysphasic children needed an undue amount of time to process longer sequences, but there was in addition the strong possibility that there was an additional independent defect of memory for temporal order. They conclude "Whatever the underlying cause, dysphasic children do *in effect* have inferior memory for auditory sequences" (Tallal and Piercy, 1978, p. 77, their italics).

Auditory and Sequential Memory in the Deaf

Conrad (1972) carried out a deceptively simple series of experiments to investigate the short-term memory of deaf children. In the two groups of alphabetic letters, B C D P T V and K N V X Y Z, different types of confusion may arise during recall. Phonological and the closely related articulatory confusion arises between the names of the letters in the first group, a familiar problem over the telephone; in the second group it is the shape or appearance of the letters which is likely to create difficulty. With hearing subjects Conrad (1964) had found that if the wrongly recalled letters are set up in the form of an error matrix, mistakes occur between letters which sound similar or are articulated similarly, *e.g.* F is reported as S, or P as B. Using many sequences of five or six letters at a time with severely deaf children he found that the errors they produced indicated there were two distinct populations. One group relied on articulatory coding for memorizing names of letters, whilst the other probably relied on their visual appearance. Because of the degree of hearing loss it was considered that neither group could rely on auditory imagery. The children who tended to resort primarily to articulatory coding correlated well with those who had been separately and independently assessed by their teachers as being the better speakers.

In a subsequent extensive study of deaf school-leavers, Conrad (1979) suggested that the short-term memory deficit traditionally reported by those who work with deaf school children probably reflected an artefact introduced by the nature of the material used by normally hearing teachers. It has long been assumed that auditory processing of speech is dependent upon a temporal sequencing ability. The corollary is that this ability must be defective in the deaf child. Conrad (ibid., p. 138) concludes that "the recall of items sequentially does not depend on normal hearing, nor on normal language ability, nor exclusively on the use of phonetic coding—but on whether coding options available to the subjects are effective for the material to be memorized".

Cognitive Function

The assumption which has provided the basis in these pages for description of the processes underlying the development of language is that the way in which the child perceives, orders and conceptualizes his world is of fundamental importance in language acquisition. If this were in fact the case it should be possible to come across children in whom there is some form of impairment of intellectual function and demonstrate the co-occurrence of impairment of spoken language. Though the argument has been developed in this way, it must be pointed out in fairness to the reader that one's own understanding of the nature of language development has followed a course which is the exact opposite of that described. Arising out of experience with children showing various types of difficulty in the acquisition of speech and language, a point of view has been reached which asserts that normally developing cognitive processes are essential to the normal acquisition of language. It is measure of the strength of the position adopted by an impressive number of psychologists and developmental psycholinguists that theoreticians and clinicians can converge to a common view-point.

The opinion of virtually anyone in the community as a whole would be that the mentally backward have problems in talking with those around them. This notion has passed into popular usage in the contemptuous undertones which accompany the word "dumb", invariably implying stupidity. Precisely the same attitude finds expression in very different cultures. In Luganda, the language of the Bantu people centred on Kampala in Uganda, *omusiru* is the noun (rarely) used in a derogatory and offensive way to mean a foolish person. From it is derived *kasiru* with the same root meaning the dumb or deaf-and-dumb. Unfortunately, neither lay nor professional wisdom is able to quantify the precise relationship between mental retardation and the ability to talk. Mittler (1972) says:

"The ability to use language is obviously closely bound up with the development of intelligence, but the relationship between them is far from simple. That a child is mentally subnormal should not be regarded as a necessary or sufficient explanation for his inability to talk ..." (p. 136)

and he goes on to point out an essential fact which is too frequently overlooked even now, that the child who is slow in learning to talk is by no means necessarily mentally backward.

The Relation Between "Intelligence" and Language Attainment

There is no simple, direct relationship between the degree of impairment of intelligence and that of spoken language. Indeed, it would be highly surprising if there were. The results of psychological assessment expressed in terms of mental age or intelligence quotient are based on scores obtained on a variety of standardized tests. These were not designed to distinguish between the innumerable forms of mental retardation, each with their particular profile of deranged neuropsychological functioning. Very different patterns of neurological pathology and cognitive dysfunction may result in the same score on an IQ scale. Based on his studies of psychotic children, Rutter (1972) considers that non-verbal performance tests are of vital importance in children who cannot speak at an age appropriate level, and that a low performance score is associated with a poor prognosis in language development. This is undoubtedly true. One also sees a number of children in whom the disturbance of language acquisition is out of all proportion to the effect of the (sometimes necessarily assumed) underlying neurological lesion on overall non-verbal intelligence.

In the personal series of 315 children already referred to, it can be seen from Table 7.4 that there is a certain correspondence between the child's ability to carry out the performance items of intelligence tests and his verbal comprehension. Discrepancies are apparent. Allowing for the differences in degree of standardization of the various types of assessment procedure and for the relatively crude indication of disability on a three point scale, there is a clear tendency for there to be more children with impairment of verbal comprehension (98) than one would expect from the results of formal psychological assessment (60). This is in accord with clinical experience, and there is no shift of the data in the reverse direction.

Table 7.4. *The relation between the child's intelligence, as measured with the non-verbal subscales of standard intelligence tests, and verbal comprehension. All children with hearing loss have been excluded*

	Verbal Comprehension			
Performance IQ	Normal	Moderate impairment	Severe impairment	Totals
Normal	76	26	13	115
Moderate impairment	1	18	7	26
Severe impairment		2	32	34
Totals	77	46	52	175

Mental Handicap and Intelligence

It is possible to recognize a number of specific conditions associated with cognitive dysfunction, such as the chromosomal abnormalities of which Trisomy 21 is the most common, being responsible for 5—10% of all mental defect (McKay, 1977), presenting clinically as Down's syndrome or mongolism. There are many other causes, of an inherited nature, or arising from damage through infections, or through antenatal hazards during the intrauterine period, or as complications of the neonatal period and later. In a large number of children it is not possible to state the cause of the mental handicap. Such a variety of causes, known and unknown, must inevitably result in a multiplicity of effects on the brain. The brain itself, whether structurally or functionally, cannot be thought of as a global whole or as a single organ. It is an immensely complicated collection of neural organs and their interconnections, the diversity of function of which is at least as great as that of the various organ systems in the thoracic and abdominal cavities. Pathological effects may be widespread or localized, particulate, microscopic or large scale; they may be confined to a certain neural system or damage many. The results may be seen in disturbances of sensory processing and motor function; at the level of ordering and organization of perception or the coordination and integration of skilled motor acts; of the systems subserving memory, alertness and attention; or of the higher orders still of cognitive function, in concept formation and the operations we carry out on these concepts; and on the modes of expression we employ to convey the results of our thinking and feeling.

The concept of intelligence, though intuitively appealing and historically important, has very little to offer the clinician and the teacher concerned with the minutiae of the individual child's pattern of cognitive assets and deficits. Intelligence tests serve on the whole as predictors of educational attainment within the community at large, and as such have a valuable role, but this is the beginning, not the end, of assessment. There needs to be a reorientation of the role of the psychologist into a close working partnership with developmental and neurological paediatrics, akin to the pathologist who measures or identifies variations of normal function whether it be the electrolyte concentrations or protein fractions of the blood, or the changes in composition of the numerous tissues of the body at a biochemical or cellular level. The logic of the belief that language is primarily and essentially the corollary of human cognitive structure (allied to the necessity for precisely modulated interaction between individuals) demands no less than that in due course of time the neuropsychological aspects of its disorders be investigated at this level of resolution.

Language Characteristics in the Mentally Handicapped

Studies of the language of subnormal children suggest that retardation does not yield a different form of language behaviour, but rather a slowing of the normal sequence of linguistic development, and a termination of development below that attained by normal children. This is the conclusion reached by Lackner (1968) in his detailed examination of the grammatical structures of 5 children. The grammars he was able to write for each of these children showed that there was spontaneous generation of sentences (a fundamental characteristic of any true language system) and that these bore an appropriate relationship to adult grammar. The differences lay in the degree of limitation, in the over-general, non-specific nature of the utterances and in their lack of sensitivity to the context in which they were produced. O'Connor and Hermelin (1963) had earlier reached the same conclusion. The results of some of their experimental investigations revealed the following:

a) The structure of language used by subnormal children resembles that of normal children at the corresponding stage of development.

b) If the severely retarded use a word in speech, it has the same semantic characteristics as for normal children at an equivalent age, and word associations to nouns fall into the same descriptive response.

c) Semantic generalization does occur in the subnormal, and the effect of this is evident in subsequent word associations.

d) The severely subnormal can use concepts as a principle of classification, though they may be unable to verbalize such concepts.

In his description of the receptive language of severely subnormal children derived from work carried out at the Hester Adrian Research Centre in Manchester, Wheldall (1976) based his findings on the use of the Sentence Comprehension Test developed by Hobsbaum and Mittler (1971). The test comprises 15 subtests in which various types of grammatical structure are used, and the child has to point to the correct one out of four pictures. A particular subtest might be centred on the understanding of an intransitive verb, the identification of plurals, or of a difficult preposition. Wheldall assessed the verbal comprehension of 86 severely subnormal children in comparison with 30 nursery school children, matched for their scores on the English Picture Vocabulary Test. The results have been rearranged into tabular form (Table 7.5) and show very close agreement between the two groups, at the equivalent mental age. Furthermore, he concluded that the development of the skills required for the comprehension of the more complex sentences kept pace with vocabulary development in the retarded children.

Table 7.5. *Comparison of abilities of 86 ESN(S) children and 30 ordinary children using the English Picture Vocabulary Test (EPVT) and the Sentence Comprehension Test (SCT) derived from Wheldall (1976)*

Category of child	CA, years	EPVT, months	SCT, score
Severely subnormal	$12^1/_2$	53	32
Nursery class	4	51	34

There are of course differences in verbal behaviour, and these have been summarized by Mitchell (1976) in his review of a number of reports in the literature. The subnormal child in comparison with the ordinary child at the equivalent stage of mental development is more unintelligible; he is less soliciting or accepting of control, meaning that he asks less questions, does not request guidance to the same extent, and is less prepared to submit his tentative ideas to adults; he is more echoic, repeating what is said to him; and in his utterances he is less likely to include tacts (*i.e.* naming, labelling or describing), mands (*i.e.* demanding, commanding, requesting) and interverbals, which are defined as responses that are under the control of verbal stimuli, but with no direct, point to point correspondence with them.

Play and Cognitive Deficit

The importance of symbolic play in the acquisition of language has already been noted. Developing a line of approach prompted by Sheridan and as outlined by Sheridan in 1968, it has been personal clinical practice since that time to use a selection of everyday household objects and types of play material not simply to facilitate communication with the child, but to assess the level of his development in this area. It is not a standardized procedure in any statistical sense, but has acquired a certain hidden formality of its own and is an invaluable tool in the evaluation of the children seen. Despite the lack of standardization it is interesting to see the relationship it reveals with verbal comprehension, Table 7.6. The inter-relationships between verbal comprehension and performance IQ, and similarly for play as shown here, reveal the same trends. There is no more than a marginal number of children performing better at verbal comprehension than in symbolic play; and as the development of comprehension falls further behind, so the grasp of the significance of the symbolic content of the play materials is reduced. There is an appreciable number of children who have a more severe deficit of comprehension relative to play (Table 7.6 17+3+17, or 21%) as there was for the performance IQ (Table 7.4 26 + 13 + 7, or 26%). There is however a definite reduction in number of the children with severe comprehension deficit reported as showing normal play (3 or 1.7%) compared with normal performance (13 or 7.4%). It should be remembered that the assessment of play, and frequently also of verbal comprehension is carried out non-formally during the course of routine outpatient clinics.

Table 7.6. *Comparison of the levels of attainment in verbal comprehension and play in 315 children. All children with hearing loss worse than 30 dB have been excluded, leaving 175 for comparison*

	Verbal Comprehension			
Level of Play	Normal	Moderate impairment	Severe impairment	Totals
Normal	69	17	3	89
Moderate impairment	7	26	17	50
Severe impairment		2	34	36
Totals	76	45	54	175

A more formally researched study of the relationship between play, retardation and verbal comprehension is that of Wing, Gould, Yeates, and Brierly (1977). Their series of 108 children included all those in a defined area of London who were attending any type of school, hospital or home for severely retarded children, and certain other categories of disability such as autism, psychosis or severe language disorder were also included. The children's ages ranged from 5—14 years, rather more than two thirds of them being 10 years old or more. It was found that no child with a non-verbal age of less than 20 months had developed symbolic play. This applied to 31 children and in all of them the level of verbal comprehension was in the 0—19 month range. There were 11 children whose non-verbal mental age was at a higher level who also failed to develop symbolic play, 6 of them having early childhood autism. Only 2 children in this group had a verbal comprehension age, as measured on the Reynell Developmental Language Scale (Reynell, 1969) above 19 months and both showed the classic autistic syndrome. There was a group of 23 children who had developed a measure of play, referred to as "stereotyped" because though there was apparently some pretend play this was restricted, repetitive and with a complete lack of innovation, rather as if a sequence had been copied and perpetuated. Almost all had non-verbal and verbal comprehension ages above 20 months. At best the children showed repetitive, stereotyped speech, sometimes with persistent questioning that was inappropriate to the situation; in many there was marked abnormality of language development. In the group of 43 children who had achieved symbolic play, at the least playing appropriately with a car or a doll, most were placed in the educational services for the severely subnormal rather than in residential units, and there was a higher proportion in this group than in the others of children with Down's syndrome. This level of play was reported as occurring in less than half of the schoolage severely retarded children.

The Importance of Pretend Play

Because of our attitudes to child play and our inability to take it seriously there is widespread difficulty in realizing that symbolic and pretend play represents a remarkable level of cognitive development. Before it can develop, people, objects of many sorts and sizes, the emergence of order in space and time, the nature of cause and effect, and all of these in their turn dependent on the adequate functioning and integration of diverse sensory and motor processes, must become real to the child. He must be able to understand each of these various features of his environment as existing and acting independently of himself, and must then be able to represent them all internally, and have recourse to them as and when he has need of them. It must be as important to remove the mental representations or images from the mind's eye when no longer required as to conjure them up on demand, and one wonders if this process of erasure can be faulty; it might be part of the explanation of highly perseverative behaviour or of stereotyped play. Symbolic play appears to be one of those step-wise jumps in human cognitive evolution, enabling us to internalize our world and act upon it, manipulating its various components (within certain limits) as we choose. The next stage is the transition from symbol to sign and the restructuring of this cognitive ability into a form which enables us to express the results of our thinking so that it can be shared with others through language.

We have seen that in the absence of symbolic play there is severe impairment of verbal comprehension. It is necessary to pursue the matter a little further and ask if impairment of other, earlier developing cognitive structures might account for the failure of play to appear, or to be severely delayed in doing so. And the answer would be that for almost all the examples given and the stages of development described in Chapter 3, one can think of instances in which a particular child showed evidence of such a phenomenon, but months or years after it appears in the ordinarily developing child. One sees children busily arranging play materials one on top of the other oblivious of their symbolic content, or putting dolls, cars, bricks and cups indiscriminately into a doll's house as if it were a cupboard. A child who has achieved the appropriate level of understanding cannot treat the materials in this cavalier way. One might see a retarded child of $3^1/_2$ years or more absorbed in a game in which she places four bricks at carefully chosen distances from each other across the floor, looks at the result and equally carefully changes the arrangement several times. In her exploration of spatial relationships she is at the stage described by Piaget as occurring sometime after the first birthday. Such observations can be made in each of the major areas of concept development he delineates.

Elements and Classes: Categorization

There are other features of cognitive behaviour which also need to be considered. Bruner (1957) considers that the learning of concepts and the use made of these concepts is one of the most elementary and general forms of cognition by which man adjusts to his environment. Concepts represent the attempt to sort objects and events into some sort of meaningful classes, and in this long drawn out process it is necessary to distinguish between instances in which a particular example is or is not a member of a certain class. Children show this in the way for instance that they line up cars, or arrange animal-toys and transport-toys into well-defined groups, even though one of the animals is the pull-along variety with wheels attached. The construction of categories of concept, and their hierarchical organization is without doubt an essential development process, abnormalities of which may lead to problems of generalization and particularity. The autistic child's distress at being given any other than his special spoon or cup, occurring long after such behaviour has disappeared in the normal child, might be an example of this. So might his desperate insistence that certain objects must be in specific locations, or perhaps this is an example of inability to develop and separate his concepts of objects and space beyond the combined "teddy-on-bed" level. In considering the need to organize the diversity of the environment and give it meaning, O'Connor and Hermelin (1963) identify our uncertainty by asking how far severely subnormal children are able to use classifying principles as a mental tool, and to what extent are they able to apply a concept which has been acquired in order to solve a subsequent problem?

Directed Attention

The control of attention is a conspicuous difficulty in many handicapped children. Cooper, Moodley, and Reynell (1978) consider that there are six stages in the normal development of attention: extreme distractibility, seen in the first year of life; and in each of the next years—concentration for some time on a task of his own; single channelled but more flexible attention, allowing a shift from task to directions under the guidance of an adult; the beginning of control by the child of his own focus of attention; two-channelled attention so that the child can, for instance assimilate verbal directions without the need to interrupt the task at hand; and finally the stage of well-established and sustained attention. Problems of attention may arise because of the pattern and style of interaction between adult and child in the early months and years of life, but in many children the cause must be intrinsic, arising sometimes for example out of neurological dysfunction as a result of intra-uterine or perinatal damage. The effect is to retard the child's cognitive development, sometimes from the very earliest days, so that even the child's interaction with his mother is prevented. The child is afforded no opportunity to observe and process his environment in tranquillity but his waking time is taken up with restless activity, anger, distress and crying. In some of these infants, calm does finally descend, and developmental progress becomes normal. The older child, flitting from object to object, and pursuing every activity only for brief periods of time, unable to concentrate on anything for long, will similarly have difficulties in learning.

Cognitive Dysfunction and Verbal Comprehension

In the severe forms of receptive language disorder, occurring in children in whom there are no complicating factors such as abnormal social interaction or mental retardation, one cannot evade the possibility of a profound disturbance of sensory function. Not only words but even their name, and the whole range of sound activity which normally conveys so much of what is going on around us seem to have no meaning or interest. The lack of response, or even of awareness of sound, is so extensively impaired that such children might best be labelled not as receptive language disorder but as showing auditory agnosia.

Case Report: **Christopher**

He has a normal elder sister who is making good progress. He was born at full term, and delivery was uneventful. His mother however had suffered from prolonged, excessive vomiting during the pregnancy and had taken Debendox throughout. He began to say one or two recognizable words at one year, and about 20 words by 18 months. The maximum vocabulary size achieved was 50 words by sometime after his second birthday, when he was already beginning to stop using several of his earlier words and he then stopped saying any words. He had never reached the stage of two-word joining. He started showing some eyeflickering and transient absences shortly after his third birthday; an EEG record at that time showed an overall pattern of immaturity with several postaural temporal spikes and some tendency for these to be generalized. Six months later the recording was normal in every respect. When seen at about that time ($3^1/_2$ years) he was a friendly child who used his voice to produce an occasional sound in which there were no true vowels and no consonants; his play was limited to showing some recognition of miniature doll's house furniture but no ability to organize it into any replica of a real life situation, and he was interested in pictures; when assessed on the Snijders-Oomen non-verbal intelligence scale his performance was at the good average level. A review assessment 15 months later by a different psychologist confirmed normal non-verbal intelligence. His concentration was poor, and he had no recognition for spoken words. The absences and eyeflickering returned at about this time and the EEG record showed many brief generalized discharges, but no temporal spikes. Initial medication tried had been phenytoin and later clonazepam but his response was poor; on this occasion sodium valproate had an apparently beneficial effect but eventually had to be stopped and nitrazepam similarly had an initial beneficial effect, but its side effects impaired his attention and learning to such an extent that he was found to be better without medication.

Overall his progress was slow and he showed a very limited ability to learn. There was limited interaction with his teachers, which was frequently confined to sitting on someone's lap, and there was no contact with other children. At $5^1/_2$ years he still showed no recognition of spoken words, though hearing tests including electrocochleography showed no loss of hearing. Visually he could identify 12 printed nouns and a few adjectives, and using the Paget Gorman Sign System he could carry out very simple requests but found it extremely difficult to use the signs to convey meaning. When 6 years old there was more evidence of progress. He was able to recognize the spoken names of perhaps six objects and responded more consistently to his name when called; he was able to identify some of the range of normal household sounds; and was trying to imitate one or two speech sounds such as "sh".

He was able to work rather better in a small group, but still responded best to one adult, needing a great deal of individual attention. Using the Paget signs, he could carry out requests such as "Give me the ball, book and car" if they were on the table in front of him, or to "Put the tree under the table". With signs the best "utterances" he could produce were "Two fish blue" or "Bus swimming come?"—meaning "Has the bus which takes us swimming come yet?" He was able to read 25 nouns, the childrens's names in his class, and a few verbs and adjectives. He could count up to five objects, his play was more imaginative and his drawing could convey for instance, a car which he had seen being loaded onto a breakdown lorry. Speech showed a limited ability to modify a vowel-like sound by altering lip posture, so producing "ooo" or "eee" or "aah"; "m" and "sh" could be formed but it was quite impossible to combine a "consonant" and a "vowel". The Paget signing system, despite his limited ability in its use, was vital to him particularly as by now he was showing a progressively increasing desire to communicate. His verbal understanding through signs was at about the level of a $2^1/_2$ year old and expression that of a 2 year old.

The more one sees of such children and gets to know them, the more one realizes that, however profound the auditory difficulty, there are problems of cognitive function which are even more serious. Since it has been emphasized that the child's performance on non-verbal intelligence tasks was age appropriate, such a remark requires justification. This is best done by reporting a personal observation. *Observation:* Christopher in his usual vague but amiable way was carrying out a number of requests which *S*, the senior speech therapist in the unit, was giving him using the Paget-Gorman sign system. It is important to note that the objects were on the table in front of him and it was his task to place one under the table, another in front of the chair or by the window, as she named the play object and where it should go. This he managed without difficulty, but there was a remarkable change when *S* reversed the procedure, and asked him to give her each object as she signed its name. His performance deteriorated immediately, and he wandered round the room in an uncertain manner picking things up and handing them to *S* which she did not accept. As he continued his wandering his eye caught the required object on top of a low cupboard, where he had placed it not long before; his expression changed immediately, he picked it up and handed it confidently to *S*.

The immediate conclusion was that this was a simple failure of memory and in a sense it was, but if the explanation is left at this level it lacks conviction. It was much more as if the child's internal representation was so ill-defined that it was only when he saw the object, that its physical re-presentation to his vision recalled the object to mind. To put it rather differently, it was as if he knew he had to look for something, but didn't know what it was until he saw it. It is difficult to interpret his difficulty unless one accepts the possibility that for him this group of play objects had not yet become fully permanent, as in the cognitive behaviour of a child under a year old with regard to the concept of objects.

It is a recurring source of surprise to see how well some children, who clearly have great difficulty in making sense of their world, can manage to attain near-normal scores on formal intelligence testing. If one had not encountered this phenomenon on numerous occasions, the observation recounted above and its possible explanation would seem ludicrous. What any test of performance must do is to present the child with specific, concrete objects in the immediate here and now. It could hardly do otherwise. But of course it can then only give information on the child's ability to perceive and order concrete materials and their relationships, and can give no indication of the extent to which the child has developed the ability to represent them internally and permanently in the absence of tactile and visual reinforcement. There is a sense in which play materials get round this difficulty. They not only have an immediate physical reality in their size, shape, colour and substance but they have a metaphysical, *i.e.* symbolic, reality; coded into this shaped substance there is something which extends and transcends the physical features and gives them a higher order of meaning. It would be invaluable for there to be developed a series of ambivalent test materials which could be sorted or arranged as items in a performance test, or in a very different way which was appropriate to their symbolic content. The value (substantial or symbolic) which the child attached to them would be represented by the way in which he handled and arranged them.

8 The Antecedents of Disorder Voice, Speech and Language

Voice

Some children are mute. Though it is an extremely rare occurrence they seem to be virtually unable to produce any sound other than the intensely emotionally motivated crying, shrieking or laughter.

Case Report: **Simon**

He was first seen at age 5 y 11 m because of his complete inability to talk. His parents described him as a secure, happy, lazy child, well behaved and invariably good-humoured. He had sat up at 7 m, but not walked until 2 y 2 m. When seen he had a variety of slight problems with gait and overall mobility, but was good with his hands; he showed impairment of symbolic play, and was assessed at between 62—70 on the non-verbal items of selected intelligence scales. He was able to hear normally as measured by pure-tone audiometry, and understood a wide variety of the simpler type of spoken request at a level appropriate to a child of 3 y. He had never produced any sounds other than crying, laughing and coughing, though he was beginning to utter an occasional "er" sound when he pointed to what he wanted. There was no structural abnormality of the speech apparatus. His tongue showed no voluntary control in the carrying out of various movements; it was broad and atonic with poor control of overall shape and mass, there was marked asymetrical movement of the two halves, and various patterns of involuntary activity. During the subsequent six years of follow-up there has been very little change in this picture. Despite being a highly communicative child, trying to express ideas and share them with others, interested in adults and enjoying the company of other children, demonstrative and affectionate, he has not extended his vocalization beyond an occasional "mm" or "aah". He developed some simple mime, but though he acquired a moderate vocabulary of Paget Gorman signs there has been minimal spontaneous use. Specialist paediatric neurological examination had failed to reveal any abnormal signs other than the immature gait and slight clumsiness, and there was no evidence of neuromuscular disease or cerebral palsy. There was no history of any significant illness. Psychiatric assessment concluded that he was "a happy child, really attached to his parents and older sister, open and affectionate to them. They in their turn treated him with a kind of half-amused tolerance and true understanding which it was considered had helped to bring out the best in him."

There are numerous children in whom the development of pre-linguistic, vocal activity is quite severely delayed. Their parents may draw attention to the lack of baby noises, and the undue length of time which elapsed before there was any spontaneous vocalization. Babble and jargon may never have appeared, or in a very limited way. In the more extreme case, the child's attempts at verbal utterances at say, 3 yr may be restricted to a short, explosive sound with a rather strangled quality and bearing a remarkable similarity to the bleat of a young lamb or deer. Within the space of this brief pulse of sound the child tries to introduce some verbal content. If, and as, speech develops the child is obliged to talk in a series of monosyllabic pulses of sound. There is a spectrum of disability from the most severe to children in whom the coordination of motor activity for the appropriate modifications of respiration and of the laryngeal and supraglottal parts of the speech apparatus is present but poor. Speech sounds are weak, and utterances are restricted in length. This may be clearly apparent in some spastic children, but there are children in whom it is not possible to demonstrate any well defined neurological deficit.

Case Report: **Susan**

When seen for the first time she was aged 4 y 9 m with a spoken vocabulary of five words. She was born at full term after an uneventful pregnancy. She had to be intubated because of breathing difficulties associated with excessive quantities of mucus and cyanotic episodes. Throughout her life she had been prone to respiratory infections and eczema. Her mother suffered from asthma as a child but there was no other relevant history, and no one else in the family had suffered from speech problems. During the first year of life she was a very quiet child, never crying and only rarely making sounds. She was a slow feeder, often choking over her feeds, and food had to be liquidized until she was $2^1/_2$ y. She sat at 1 y, was crawling by her second birthday, stood at $2^1/_2$ y, and was walking shortly before her third birthday. She was a happy, amenable child, friendly and cooperative with strangers. Her spoken vocabulary consisted of "da" (doll), "ba" (boy), "le" (lady), "ba" (bed), "bu" (spoon), and some sounds for animals. Verbal comprehension and non-verbal intelligence were at the same level and appropriate to a child of $3^1/_2$ y when formally assessed shortly after her first visit. She had a number of difficulties arising out of impaired motor control affecting her standing posture and stability, in getting on and off chairs, and in manipulation and various self-help skills. This was subsequently attributed to a minor, ataxic cerebral palsy, with no evidence of cerebellar involvement. Her lips were open and permanently wet, there was gross

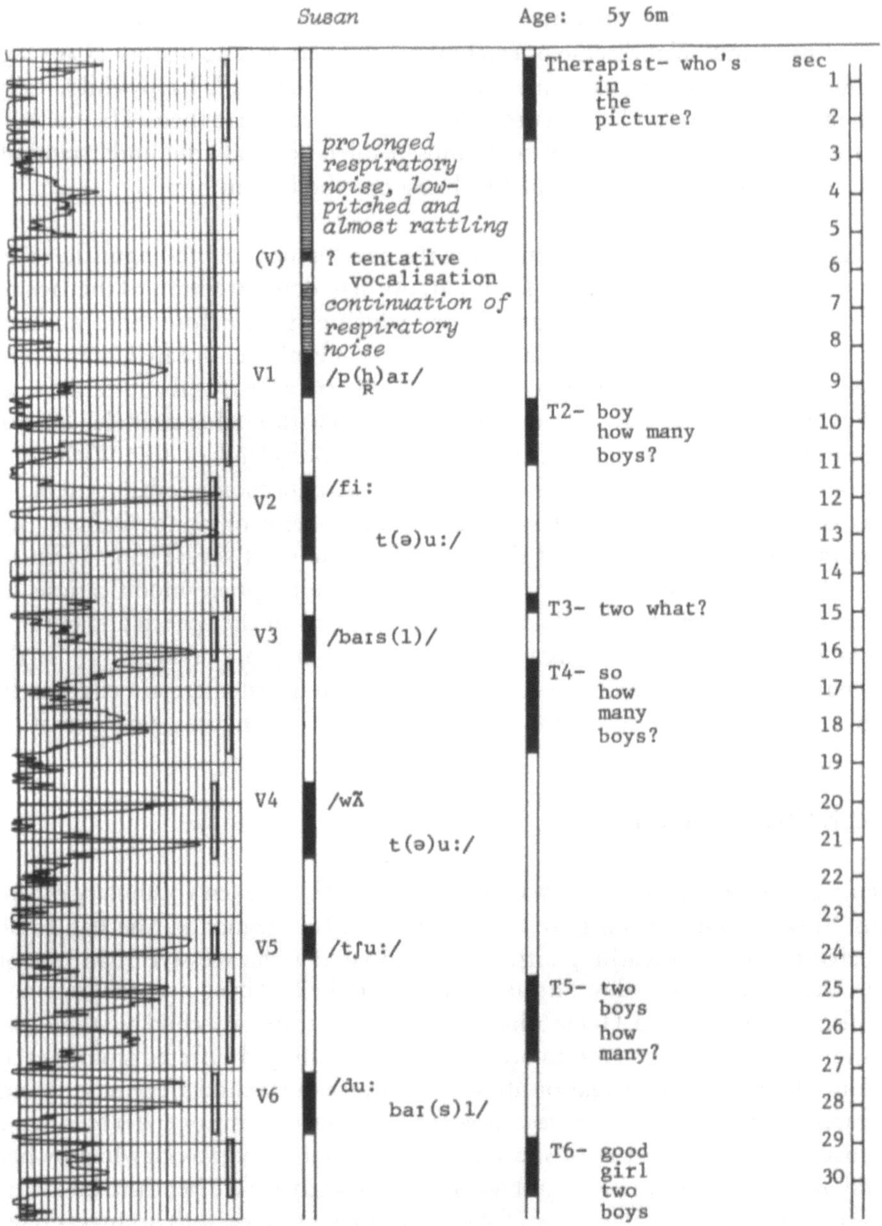

Fig. 8.1. There is prolonged, noisy respiratory activity and possibly a tentative vocalization following the speech therapist's question at T1. The child requires virtually 6.0 sec from her first audible response before she is able to produce her over-loud, single-pulsed reply. Even then the vocal apparatus is not fully under control, and there is marked palato-pharyngeal vibration, indicated by the /ʀ/ trill subscript. Her linguistic output is grossly restricted by the inability to produce more than two syllables in an utterance, and these are invariably explosive and brief. Articulatory difficulties arising from poor control of tongue and lips can be seen in the three variants of "two" at V2 (and V4), V5 and V6; and the three variants of "boy(s)" at V1, V3 and V6

limitation of voluntary control of tongue movement, and its overall shape and posture were similarly poorly controlled. She could, very carefully and deliberately, imitate a small number of speech sounds. Control of breathing for vocal activity was notably poor, so that often she could only produce one syllable per breath, taking 1—2 sec for each vocal utterance, see Fig. 8.1. Her best achievement was a maximum of two words, each of two syllables and barely intelligible, one year after she had started therapy. A further six months later by which time she was 6 y old, and after she had been receiving intensive speech therapy with particular reference to her breathing and control of the vocal carrier wave, she could sustain an utterance for 6—7 sec without needing to take a breath, and was able to articulate six syllables in an utterance.

It is on the basis of such observations that one is forced to the conclusion that there may be a primary failure of development of the carrier wave for spoken language, quite separate and distinct from articulation or "speech" problems and from specific impairment of language production. Early vocal activity is without doubt the product of an innate neurological mechanism, as was discussed in Chapter 4. This innate activity develops into the exquisitely controlled carrier wave, with its intricate modulations of pitch, volume and rhythm which characterize the vocal behaviour of the one-year-old. If it is to do so, it is necessary for the child to be able to hear the voices of competent speakers of his mother tongue, and for him to be able to hear and so to model his vocal activity until it is an acceptable approximation to theirs. Deaf children show wide variation in development of the speech carrier wave. This cannot simply be accounted for by the degree of hearing loss, and there is poor correlation between the two, even in those children who have been diagnosed and fitted with hearing aids before the first birthday. If the development of vocal activity were entirely innate up until repetitive babble of the "consonant-vowel" type, then it could be argued that provision of hearing aids at 8—9 months would ensure the smooth progression of the speech carrier wave into the long strings of jargon characteristic of a few months later. One's experience is that this happens more as the exception than the rule. The handicap of the deaf child is by no means restricted to severe language dysfunction; in many the ability to control the basic features of intonation, of duration and rhythm of "syllables" is no less defective. If one accepts the proposition that the child begins to model his vocal activity on the voices of those around him from soon after birth, it would seem likely that the deaf child's speech problems arise very much earlier than is generally accepted. Evidence in support of this view is seen in Fig. 8.2, showing the characteristics of the vocal activity of a girl child, aged 8.4 M, taken from a recording made on the day she was diagnosed deaf.

Case Report: **Anna**

Seen first at 8.4 M, she was the fourth child in the family. Her mother had contracted rubella from one of her older children when 16 weeks pregnant. Development was normal in every respect, and she was a healthy child except that she was not responding to sound. Her mother considered that her vocalization was no different from her three elder daughters at the same age. Free field testing, using localization of the sound source as the response, revealed a hearing loss of 90 dB for the usual range of test sounds, confirmed when she was 13 months old. At that time her threshold for narrow band noise stimuli in free field was 80 dB in the lower frequencies, and 90 dB for 1 kHz–4 kHz. Her vocalizations, far from being normal, were thin and tremulous, with no modulation of pitch and no complexity of temporal pattern, sufficient evidence in itself to indicate the possibility of deafness. She was fitted with a Philips 8146 hearing aid within a fortnight of her first visit. Fig. 8.3 shows a typical section from a recording made some four months after she had started wearing hearing aids. The unduly simple vocal utterances are being replaced by more complex patterning of the vocal carrier wave with respect to pulse structure, varia-

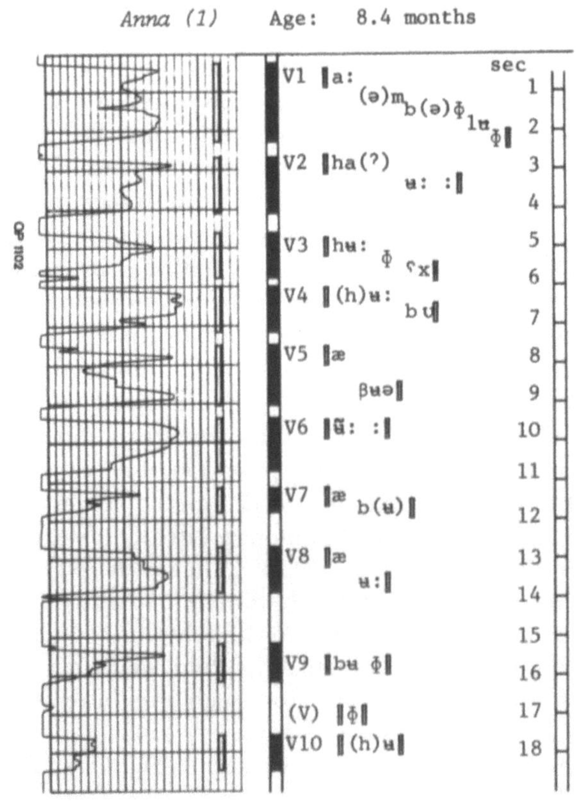

Fig. 8.2. It is remarkable that despite severe hearing loss (see text) she is spontaneously producing sounds in which there is variation of the basic pulsed structure (*e.g.* V1, V5, V8) and of the phonants themselves. An initial reaction of the listener could easily be that she is vocalizing normally. There is however a markedly deviant quality about her vocalization which renders labelling of the different sounds so difficult one cannot always be certain of the distinction between vocant and closant sounds. Because of these abnormal features it is not easy to equate the vocal activity with any particular age range. The best approximation is to that of Rosi when aged 3.5 months (p. 70), her velar "gh" /ɣ/ sounds being replaced by Anna with the bilabial "bh" /β/ and "ph" /ɸ/ sounds, perhaps because the child can see lip movement easily and so uses it herself

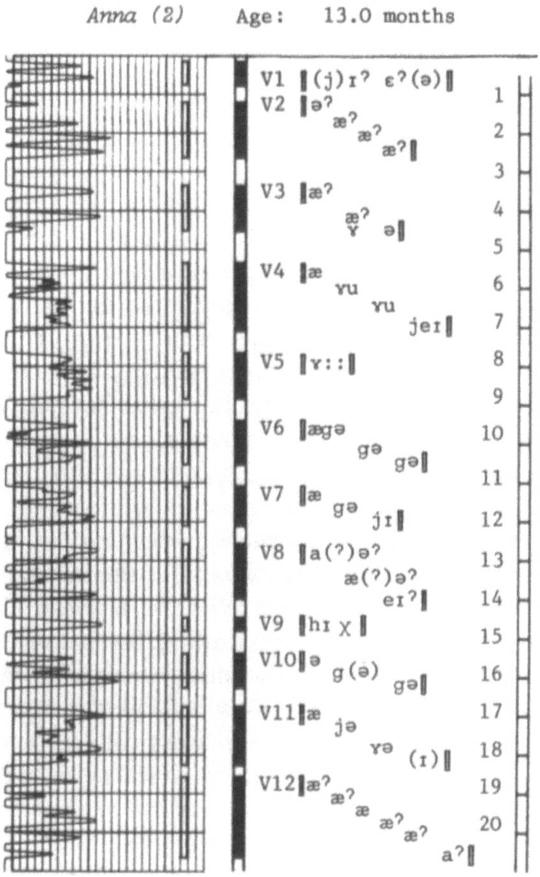

Fig. 8.3. After an interval of four months there is a marked change in her vocalization, hopefully because of the hearing-aids she has been wearing since the time of the previous recording. The trace shows two predominant vocal behaviours. In V2 and V3, and reappearing at V12, there are emphatic, staccato pulses of vocant sound, the number of pulses ranging from 3 to as many as 6. These sounds are rather harsh in quality and with minimal variation of pitch. The other behaviour may be identified at V4, V6 and elsewhere—velar "g" or "gh" sounds are introduced to produce VCVCVCV patterns of alternating vocant and closant segments. Her vocalization may be most readily equated with that of Helen at 4.5 months (p. 72), though without the variation in pitch

tions of pitch and loudness, and alternating vocant and closant sounds, as she starts to respond to these basic characteristics in the speech of her family.

Control of the voice may show more subtle disturbances which are easily overlooked. Numbers of children have a rather rough quality to the voice; inevitably one dismisses this as the result of an upper respiratory infection, probably associated with slight inflammation and oedema of the vocal folds. It is only after one has seen the child on a number of subsequent occasions, at various times of the year, and there has on most of these occasions been no evidence of infection, that realization dawns. The origin of the vocal roughness, rarely severe enough to be labelled hoarseness, and often found in association with a low-pitched voice with limited control of intonation patterns, is more probably neuromotor than inflammatory. It is hardly surprising that in some children there should be imperfect control of laryngeal activity. The length, mass and tension of each vocal fold must be perfectly matched to its opposing partner, and they must meet precisely in the midline during the adduction phase of each laryngeal cycle. It is perhaps surprising that this imperfect coordination is not seen more frequently and is relatively unimportant, except in the child who becomes frankly hoarse and in whom direct laryngoscopy reveals marked oedema and actual nodules on the vocal folds.

That a neuromotor basis seems to provide the most reasonable explanation for this sort of dysphonia is based on observations made during the course of direct laryngoscopy in infants with more extreme forms of impaired laryngeal control. Examination of a small series of children presenting with congenital laryngeal stridor revealed the probable nature of the condition to be neurological rather than structural in origin. There appeared to be incorrect coordination of activity of the muscle groups arranged around the laryngeal inlet in relation to the phases of respiration (Martin, 1963). In a quite separate group (which was not reported) a small number of neonates had respiratory obstruction which necessitated tracheostomy. Early removal of the tube was not possible and as the normal airway remained inadequate, direct laryngoscopy was repeated once or twice. This revealed what conceptually at that time was a surprising finding. Instead of there being (say) a fixed paralysis of the right vocal fold, subsequent examination might reveal that it was now the left side, or perhaps both folds, which failed to move. This could only be explained in terms of impaired control mechanisms at a more central level, rather than damage or malfunction to one recurrent laryngeal nerve in the peripheral part of its course. Less severe, and more numerous, forms of imperfect intra-laryngeal coordination are a logical corollary of these extreme clinical conditions. Fourcin (1978) from his work on the analysis of electro-laryngograph recordings concludes that laryngeal vibration in the first weeks after birth is not always well defined and regular.

Speech

There are a number of conditions which affect articulation. Ingram (1972) has developed a classification in which he distinguishes between isolated structural defects of teeth, lips, tongue, palate or related parts; disease of related structures; disproportion between different parts of the articulatory apparatus; and neurological disease which impairs the control of voluntary movement of the articulatory apparatus during speech. He defines dysarthria as defective articulation which is attributable to disorders of structure or function arising in these various ways. Clefts of the lip and palate and dental mal-occlusion are well-known structural defects. Amongst the neurological causes bilateral cerebral lesions are especially likely to affect speech, and virtually all patients who suffer from bilateral hemiplegia show dysarthria. In choreo-athetoid (or dyskinetic) cerebral palsy he has found the main cause of dysarthria to be involuntary movement of the lips, tongue or palate; whilst in the ataxic form there is weakness and incoordination of movements of these parts. Overall he concludes that 50% of cerebral palsied children have speech defects which are severe enough to impair their ability to communicate. Foley (1977) summarizes the position by saying that speech problems are found in the majority of children with athetoid cerebral palsy, in one half of the children with ataxia, and in about one-third of the diplegic. In Chapter 6 the number of children suffering with speech defects arising from cerebral palsy was seen to be about 1 per 1000 children, excluding those who in addition are mentally subnormal. It will be recalled that the prevalence of defects of speech and language amongst children entering ordinary schools is some 40—50 times higher. This latter is clearly a large and important group of children and it is necessary to look more closely into the possible antecedents of their difficulty.

In the series of 315 children there were 107 in whom hearing and non-verbal comprehension were within normal limits. Of these 107, there were 64 whose verbal comprehension was also normal but who had defective speech. There are so many aspects to speech that it is all too easy to overlook its most basic element. However profound the intellectual content of a verbal utterance and however moving its emotional force, speech activity is ultimately reduced to trains of impulses along the peripheral nerves which innervate the muscles of respiration, the larynx, the pharynx, those acting on the lower jaw, or contained in the lips, the palate and the tongue. We have already considered certain aspects of control of production of the voice, which provides the medium, or carrier wave on which the articulators can act. These are all situated in the supra-glottal part of the speech apparatus, and are ideally placed to modify the flow of pulsed sound coming from the larynx, and in doing so to impart special characteristics of their own. Movements of individual parts may be defective, such as the lips or the soft palate. It is no accident, but an expression of the deep, intuitive understanding of the situation that the words for "language" and for "tongue" are virtually synonymous in many European and other languages. We would have saved ourselves and our child-patients much misunderstanding if we had listened more closely to the voice of folklore, and looked more closely at this remarkable structure. The motor skills which the young child has to acquire by the age of 2—3 years in the use of her tongue rival those of any highly skilled adult in the physical execution of his craft, whether it be the playing of a musical instrument, a surgeon operating on the ossicles of the middle ear, or a professional sportsman.

The Tongue

The tongue needs to be understood in three-dimensional terms, as occupying volume or space. This in itself is difficult because one normally only sees the tip and some part of the upper surface. It is essentially a (fairly) homogeneous mass of muscle tissue which lies along the midline of the floor of the mouth, but which is composed functionally of two separate muscle masses, bilaterally symmetrical, and each with its own nerve supply. The tongue can alter in shape so that it may be pointed, thin and elongated beyond the incisor teeth, it may be retracted and squat, lying in a contracted mass on the floor of the mouth, or it may bulge smoothly upwards and backwards into the back part of the mouth cavity. It may be hard and tense, or atonic and flop over the lower teeth and lip. At rest it may be still, but never normally totally quiescent, it may be completely inert or show a variety of involuntary activity. This latter may take the form of overall twisting or writhing of the tongue along its long axis, or there may be sudden episodes of shortening in which the tongue tip appears as if it has been removed; or the involuntary activity may take a different form and appear as ripples, often quite marked and more like waves, of contraction spreading along the tongue from its posterior third, or starting at the sides and moving to the midline. The child may have the greatest difficulty even in putting the tip of the tongue out of his mouth, and there may be a variety of involuntary movements of its body as he tries this. It may be extremely difficult for him to locate particular points along his upper or lower lip, or to touch individual teeth identified for him by the clinician with a probe. In some children who show this type of difficulty it is oversimplifying the issue simply to regard it as a problem in motor control, and there may be sensory impairment, either of tactile sensation in the oral mucosa or teeth, or possibly in the feedback mechanisms from the tongue musculature.

Neuro-Motor Dysfunction

If one examines the tongue whilst it is carrying out sound-producing activity, the tongue may be positioned incorrectly or its shape may be wrong for certain sounds. Even for the longer, more steady-state production of vowel-like sounds the tongue may constantly be moving around, with unequal contraction of the two longitudinal halves. Repetitive movements for producing a series of "d-d-d-d" or "k-k-k-k" sounds may not be possible, or if the child succeeds, he may be quite unable to combine two sound elements into a pattern such as "d-g-d-g-d-g". That this control problem is not restricted to the tongue but is more widespread may be shown by the child having difficulty in producing a pattern of sound such as "b-b-b-b" or "b-d-b-d", in which lip movement is required. It is then necessary to watch the child as he tries to say simple words in which the same combination of sounds occurs, or any words which he can say easily even if inaccurately. Oral, speech and verbal dyspraxias (the terminology is unsatisfactory) are much more common than is generally realized, as revealed by the difficulties children show in trying to carry out these types of manoeuvre. Dyspraxia is used here in the sense it is used by Johns and La Pointe (1976). The term directs attention to the motor aspects of speech; it emphasizes the volitional execution of articulation; it excludes significant weakness, paralysis and incoordination of the speech musculature; and it indicates a discrepancy between the execution of the speech act and relative linguistic intactness. As we shall see later this latter may or may not be demonstrable. They label the condition "apraxia of speech".

There are a number of reasons why these various disturbances of motor function are so often overlooked, or more surprisingly their existence denied. It is characteristic of many such impaired motor processes in the developing child that they may be clearly apparent one day, and yet on another occasion there may be no evidence of their presence; one's own clinical case-notes provide frequent evidence of this. The younger the child the more difficult it is to see unusual patterns of motor activity especially if below $2^1/_2$, quite apart from the problems of ensuring an adequate level of cooperation. There are special visuo-perceptual problems, arising from the limited view one is able to obtain and relating this picture to activity in other parts of the tongue; it requires considerable experience of the normal; and there is the mundane but crucial issue of adequate illumination. But probably the most important factor is the conceptual one, of being prepared to accept that such disturbances can occur, and to look carefully and routinely for them. Even then problems remain. A child with a severe speech defect may have no difficulty in carrying out individual movements on request, but find it an impossible task to alternate two sounds, or perhaps more puzzling, some children may not be able to carry out this latter but show very little in the way of defective speech. These and other problems of interpretation are frequently encountered, and it is only by the painstaking collection of observations that we will begin to understand their true significance.

Reference has already been made to the controversy between those who do not consider auditory perceptual factors important in an understanding of impaired language acquisition and those who do. The problem recurs in efforts to explain the faulty production of speech. If there is loss of hearing or if there is some deficit of auditory processing which leads to impaired verbal comprehension then it is reasonable to infer that this will distort the child's perception of speech and result in defective speech as he tries to reproduce what he has misheard. In children who have no difficulty in identifying words correctly, and who furthermore are able to understand all that is said to them at an age-appropriate level (as applies to the 64 out of 315 children presently being considered) there are marked objections to the view that perceptual problems are the cause of the defective speech. Perceptual difficulties are present without a doubt, and it is important to appreciate their significance in the various phonological disturbances of child speech, but they frequently arise out of these defects rather than cause them. A child of 5 or 6 years may find it totally beyond his power to produce a particular phoneme, say /g/, in speech even when he can manage it in isolation. He can perceive the difference between it and the sound he habitually substitutes in its place, say /d/, and has no difficulty in carrying out the necessary discriminations in the speech of others. But he himself has been perpetuating this error ever since he first encountered difficulty in articulating "g" perhaps 3 years previously and developed his own articulatory, speech-motor solution. He has been living with a perceptual mismatch for all this time between the way he hears himself say the relevant words, and the way he hears everyone else say them.

Spoken Language

Case Report: **Felicity**

She was first seen at the age of 5 y 10 m because of severe limitation of speech. Pregnancy, birth and development were normal with the exception of her speech. There had been limited vocalization in infancy, she began to say one or two words shortly after her first birthday, and her vocabulary had increased to 20—30 "words" by the age of 2. Word-joining occurred before the end of the ensuing year. By this time she was becoming very frustrated and depressed because of her difficulties, and crying in her sleep. Despite this her parents described her as being a happy child by nature, with good comprehension. Assessment confirmed her ability to understand spoken language at a level appropriate to her age. She had a large vocabulary, and was probably putting a number of words together; a parental example was "Mum... Dad... going... round... back". Those who did not know her found her speech extremely difficult to understand, and her parents themselves found that there was considerable variation in the clarity of her speech. She had an extremely limited phonological system. The sound contrasts she used were "b", "m", an "m"-like sound produced without laryngeal voicing as a puff of air through the nose whilst she kept her lips closed, and a glottal stop. There were two vowels. With these few sounds she had developed a formal, stereotyped system which enabled her to communicate with those who knew her, and she was highly vocal, using her voice all day long. She had a squint, and her face was rather blank, with only slight movements of the lips, cheeks and forehead; she tended either to look very solemn or to laugh, and was unable to smile. There was virtually no voluntary control of the substance of the tongue, which showed a variety of patterns of involuntary activity. Hearing was normal. The sound system she had developed reveals the remarkably skilful and tenacious way by which she had tried to circumvent the gross problems of neuromotor control in the speech apparatus.

Up to this point we have been careful to identify and maintain a distinction between speech and language, the former relating to the sounds of speech and the manner of their production, and "language" referring to the content or meaning of what is said and the rules governing sentence construction, word order, verb inflections and so on. The problems of terminology of vocal activity in the prelinguistic child (Chapter 4) showed implicitly that any such clear-cut distinction between the concepts of speech and language was extremely difficult to sustain. It was found necessary to develop a descriptive vocabulary of terms for the sounds produced by the young child which are distinct from the terms describing sound production once words, in their full linguistic sense, come into use. In other words, terms like "vowel", "consonant" and "syllable" can only be used to describe linguistic phenomena and it becomes meaningless to preserve the distinction between speech and language beyond a certain point, a point which is conceptually near at hand rather than being remote or irrelevant.

The issue is an important one in considering certain patterns of expressive language disorder. In the series of 315 children, there were 47 children with moderate

Table 8.1. *Relation between language production and speech in 47 children with normal comprehension, hearing and non-verbal cognition*

	Speech		
Language Production	Normal	Moderate impairment	Totals
Moderate impairment	7	16	23
Severe impairment	5	19	24
Totals	12	35	47

or severe impairment of verbal expression in whom verbal comprehension, hearing, non-verbal performance and symbolic play were all within normal limits. The various combinations of impaired performance in speech and language production are shown in Table 8.1. Results of the type of analysis reported here need to be viewed with caution. Anyone who has had experience of children with disorders of verbal expression knows how difficult it is to achieve any accuracy of linguistic assessment when much of what the child says is unintelligible. Two words might be discernible in a flow of speech-like sound in which it is impossible to identify any further verbal items. Is this child at the stage of one-word or two-word utterances and producing strings of jargon, or is this a gross under-estimate of his language production? It is frequently possible to decide that a child's linguistic level is age appropriate, as in the 29 children shown in Tab. 7.3; it is equally possible to decide in some children that language production is impaired and there are no accompanying deficits of speech, as in the 12 children in Table 8.1. There are numerous instances, typified by the 35 children in this same table in whom it is difficult to decide whether the fault is primarily "speech" or "language" in origin. The subsequent progress of the child under therapy will frequently help decide the issue: for instance a child who has a significant problem in the neuromotor control of some aspects of speech-sound production may show remarkable gains in linguistic production as he is enabled to articulate the sounds correctly and at the proper rate. In other children it is not possible to resolve the question in this way. It becomes clear in them that the question is no longer appropriate, but that the problem has been misrepresented through the over-use of the speech versus language dichotomy. There is another approach to the problem.

Phonological Disorder

It is possible to classify all the phonemes, or linguistically meaningful sounds in a given language through certain characteristics such as whether laryngeal activity resulting in voicing is present or not; whether the sounds do or do not show frication, as in "f" versus "p"; the place of origin in the vocal tract, and certain other features. This was done for instance by Miller and Nicely (1955) who produced a classification of certain of the English consonants. The classic attempt to carry out an analysis of this type, but far wider ranging in its scope and implications, is that of Jakobson, as described for instance in Jakobson, Fant, and Halle (1952). Phonemes are the sounds in a language which serve to contrast one word and its meaning from another word. If as happens in some Bantu languages there is no distinction between "l" and "r" the two sounds can be used interchangeably with no alteration in meaning of the word, and in this instance the two are examples of one phoneme. English has a number of different ways of producing certain sounds such as "l", or "k", which are all classed together so that there is only one "l" or one "k" phoneme, but this might not be the case in some other languages. The sounds used in speech cannot be considered apart from their use in words. Though a phoneme may be defined as the smallest unit of speech that distinguishes one word from another, it can be seen that each phoneme is not an indivisible unit but is composed of a number of features. If there is to be a minimal but significant distinction between two speech sounds, Jakobson and his co-writers consider that the listener is faced with a two-choice situation in which that feature either is or is not present.

"The choice between the two opposites may be termed *distinctive feature.* The distinctive features are the ultimate entities of language since no one of them can be broken down into smaller linguistic units. The distinctive features combined into one simultaneous or ... concurrent bundle form a phoneme." (ibid. p. 3)

These features might be for instance "consonantal" or "nasal" or "continuant" out of a total list of twelve, and are either present or not present. The relevance of this to child development is that Jakobson considers the child does not acquire a list of phonemes as such, but his phonology develops in an orderly fashion dependent on his ability to perceive and use distinctive features. This acquisition is based on a hierarchical scheme in which certain contrasts must be acquired before others, *i.e.* consonants versus vowels before nasals versus orals before dental versus labial consonants and so on (Jakobson and Halle, 1968). These features build up into phonemes and they in their turn form syllables. "The pivotal principle of syllable structure is the contrast of successive features within the syllable" (p. 422). The ordering of sounds in syllables and words is a basic characteristic of speech, and it is clear that the child must learn a series of rules which govern the possible sequences of phonemes. Some sounds are frequently found in "ordered pairs", as it were, whilst other combinations cannot occur in a particular language.

This process of acquiring the phonological system of the language may well account for some of the difficulties encountered by children. If the child has normal comprehension, it would seem possible to exclude any problem of the perceptual processing of speech. On the productive side, though neuromotor problems in the articulation of speech sounds and of sequences of sound are common, it cannot be maintained that this is the only antecedent of so-called speech defects. "Articulation" should be considered as having two components. There is the motor skill in producing the sounds at the right place in the right manner at the proper rate; and there is also the cognitive, or more precisely the specifically linguistic knowledge relating to the possible juxtapositions and sequences of the sounds comprising syllables and words. Where this latter is defective, the child has a phonological disorder. The way in which this might arise is shown by the results of experimental testing of some hypotheses relating to perception and production in child phonology reported by Edwards (1974). In considering the acquisition by the child of certain contrasting features it was postulated for instance that children would first perceive the adult's "s" and "sh" as "s", and so would inevitably pronounce these two sounds as "s". In the next stage perception of the two would be accurate, but production would not differentiate between the two; after a further stage in which "sh" might at times be produced either as "s" or "sh", the child would produce the sounds correctly as he said the words that contained them. For this particular contrast the data supported the hypothesis, but this was not always the case. It may also be noted, as others have done, that her findings give a strong measure of support to Jakobson's and Halle's theory concerning the order of acquisition of distinctive features, and so of types of phoneme, but in various particular instances there were significant exceptions.

Language Production

If we turn now to words themselves rather than the sounds of which they are composed, and consider the ways in which there may be disturbances of language production we find the same types of difficulty occurring but at a higher level of organization. It may seem surprising that a child can be normal in every respect, with no hearing loss, no demonstrable impairment of any aspect of cognitive function, and verbal comprehension which is at least age appropriate (and in some children may be above average), yet have difficulties in language production. Nevertheless this is a not infrequent occurrence, as seen in Table 8.1. There are moderately retarded children in the same predicament, with deficits of language production which are in excess of their impaired cognitive function and verbal comprehension. This applied to 16 of the 315 children, but the figure fails to give an adequate indication of the true prevalence of the condition, which is almost certainly much higher than presently realized.

The ways in which language production may be impaired are probably as many as the various developmental levels and forms of linguistic expression, of clause and phrase structure, of the different parts of speech, and the morphological structure and grammatical modifications of words. The appearance of the first words may be delayed by months or years, even in the absence of impaired speech mechanisms which might render the utterances unintelligible. Vocabulary growth thereafter may be surprisingly quick, or the very much slower rhythm of development compatible with this late appearance of words may be retained. One feature seen not infrequently in retarded children is the reported appearance of words at about the appropriate time or not long thereafter, only to find that the words are not retained and are no longer used. This frequently gives rise to the conclusion that something special happened at that time which caused the child to stop talking. It is not difficult in any family to find some event which might plausibly serve as an emotional bar to further communication, whether it be the arrival of another child, an accident of some sort, or illness involving someone in the family; or parents might take the guilt upon themselves and find some cause in their own behaviour. On the other hand, it is sometimes thought to be evidence of a progressive brain lesion, despite the lack of supporting evidence of other neurological signs. In many such children one cannot deny that words did appear, but with the evidence of retardation, the probable explanation is that the words were not being used in any linguistic or meaningful sense, but were the imitation of words said to the child or in his vicinity. Some "words", so-called, are in fact only said once or twice and disappear, sometimes to be replaced by other "words" on the same transient basis. Some words become the equivalent of stereotyped gestures and are uttered for no apparent reason in a variety of situations, or the child may simply give up the imitation of word-sound until he has developed the necessary cognitive skills which enable him to make proper use of words.

In some children there is an undue delay before the appearance of word joining. Long after the stage of vocabulary size has been reached when the ordinary child has begun to produce two-word utterances, he continues to use single words though the number of words in his vocabulary may amount to 80 or in some children, many more. This seems to be a very different type of language deficit and suggests a different type of linguistic process from that of labelling and single-word utterances. Despite the normally smooth transition from one-word to two- to three- and more word utterances this does not mean that the same linguistic processes are operating. Clinical evidence suggests an alternative possibility, that there are a number of discontinous linguistic processes. In the normal child these overlap and enable her to make progress in what appears to be linear fashion up a slope, whereas it should probably be conceived as a series of steps up a staircase of increasing complexity. In children in whom there is delay in word-joining, it is often found that there is an undue preponderance of names or labels for objects and there is no means of indicating activity or relationship between objects, whether these be human or inanimate. Many deaf children in the 8—10 y range and older seem to be trapped in the earliest stages of language development as far as spoken language is concerned, using words syntactically in a way appropriate to a child of perhaps 2 years. This is not to be confused with the child's language abilities as revealed in other modalities such as the use of manual forms of communication in the various sign languages or in his ability to read and write. He may in this way have three separate "language ages", oral, manual and written, depending on his hearing loss and the effectiveness of his hearing aids, and the efficacy of the various forms of verbal (though not necessarily spoken) communication which are used to convey language and make it available to him.

As the child begins to put more words together, other difficulties may appear. These might relate to the use of prepositions, or the various forms of personal and possessive pronouns; there might be difficulties in the use of the auxiliary verb forms relating to "is" or "have" or "do", and in the formation of past and future tenses. Word order may be wrong, or words completely omitted, or the child may be unable to apply the rules which change the order of words in questions such as "Can I do it?" There may be an overall lack of questioning and in particular, questions using the WH words, who?, when?, and the more advanced how? and why? may not be used, or appear at a very much later stage. In some children the words uttered may be clearly recognizable if taken as individual items in a string, but the utterance as a whole may be quite unintelligible because of the absence of underlying linguistic structure. It then becomes impossible for the listener to abstract any meaning from the flow of words, properly articulated though each one is. Other children have a different type of problem, in which it is not so much the syntax which is at fault but the difficulties the child has in finding and using certain words, so that alternative, but in the particular context only marginally appropriate words may be uttered. Many children with expressive problems can appear to be reasonably fluent when they are able to talk about concrete objects and events taking place in their immediate here and now. But when the discussion becomes slightly more generalized and abstract their performance falls off sharply and they are unable to sustain any sort of conversation however simple, at this level.

Case Report: **Jeremy**

He was first seen at the age of 5 y 11 m, his parents being deeply concerned over his spoken language and his progress at school. His teachers had found similar difficulties and he had been referred for psychological assessment. Testing him on the Wechsler Primary and Pre-School Inventory had revealed a performance IQ of 114, and a verbal IQ of 95. When seen it was clear that the test results failed to convey the nature and extent of his problem. First words had appeared at about 1 year, but he was slow in talking and word joining had not occurred until long after his second birthday. Although at the time of his first visit he appeared to be fluent and to talk easily, the impression was erroneous. He had very limited grasp of linguistic structure for sentence formation and was not accurate beyond the stage of expanded subject-verb-object sentences, corresponding to Stage IV of the Crystal schema of syntactic analysis (Crystal *et al.*, 1976). There were numerous errors relating to the choice of individual words, of verb tenses and of word order so that it could be very difficult to understand what he was trying to say. He had difficulty in explaining things and no doubt it was this that made his teachers think that there were learning problems. He would produce an accurate description of a picture *e.g.* "That's a postman delivering letters" but might follow this with a quite inadequate attempt for another picture, *e.g.* "Boy picking up something", the something being clearly apparent. His difficulties became more obvious when he was expected to participate in a more abstract type of conversation when there were no immediate objects or events to which he could refer directly. On being asked what he liked doing at school he replied "I like doing my news writing . . ." After a brief, encouraging question he continued "What I done at home . . .", and a further prompt elicited "I done it". These clinic observations were not the stilted utterances of a child in unfamiliar surroundings but were entirely consistent with the difficulties his parents had been concerned about at home. With speech therapy specifically designed to help him develop the necessary linguistic structures, the complexity of his sentences began to increase *e.g.* "Cos the little ones get falled over and kicked" though he continued to have word finding difficulties and grammatical errors were numerous. Verbal comprehension was age appropriate. Additional help was then provided in the form of participation in a remedial group once a week and by the time he had reached 7 y 3 m there had been marked improvement, so that he could produce long expressive sentences without errors. Concurrently with this improvement his demeanour changed, he was more self-assured and prepared to take the initiative, could manage well at school and his appetite was better.

Familial and Hereditable Factors

It may be possible to identify the cause of handicap in some children. There may be other evidence of a specific, genetically determined condition; it may be possible to attribute the cause to an intrauterine infection such as rubella; or there may have been particular hazards encountered by the child during the birth process, in the neonatal period or during subsequent development. It has long been accepted that in many deaf children there is no detectable cause. In the study of hearing-impaired children in the European Community, no less than 44% of 3359 children were labelled "Cause Unknown". As Fraser (1976) has suggested, it is probable that the majority of children with a sensorineural deafness in whom it is not possible to identify the cause of the lesion are the outcome of a genetic, recessively determined disorder.

The child with some form of disorder of spoken language in the absence of deafness, mental handicap or other clearly apparent associated condition is even more of an enigma. Only on rare occasions is it possible to identify a cause, and the majority of investigations, biochemical, electroencephalographic and other fail to offer any insight into the pathogenesis. Nevertheless there is strong clinical

Table 8.2. *Family history and sex distribution*

Category of disorder		Positive family history							Negative family history		
		N	B	G	%	S	M	F	B	G	R
I	Sensori-neural deafness	110	8	4	11	1	13	3	55	43	1.3
II 1	Speech defect only	29	14	4	62	10	8	16	8	3	4.6
2a	Language production (comprehension normal)	12	1	1	17	2	1	3	6	4	1.4
b	Language production and speech (comprehension normal)	35	11	2	37	8	7	10	17	5	4.0
3a	Verbal comprehension	11	2	1	27	2	3	—	8	—	10.0
b	Verbal comprehension and speech	20	5	5	50	7	6	7	9	1	2.3
Total (II)		107	33	13	43	29	24	34	48	13	3.1

N total number of children with the condition (all with normal intelligence)
B boys G girls
% percentage of children with a positive family history for the condition
S number of siblings affected
M, F number of relatives on the mother's side and the father's side in whom there is some history of late talking or speech difficulty (or of deafness for the deaf children)
R overall sex ratio, B : G (G=1)

evidence to support the possibility of some subtle transmissible neurological disorder as being implicated in many of these children. It has long been known that there is a marked preponderance of boys showing speech and language problems. Additional support is provided for a probable constitutional basis in many of these children by noting the occurrence of "speech difficulty", past or continuing, in other members of the family. The data on sex ratio and family history gained from the study of the 315 children are summarized in Table 8.2. The sex ratio for the deaf children may be compared with that for the deaf children in the European Community (CEC, 1980) which showed a male : female ratio of 1.2 : 1. If one restricts the search to those children with normal hearing and normal intelligence there is evidence of other members of the family being involved in 43%. As it stands this is rather circumstantial evidence for a hereditable aetiology, but the figure is surprisingly high, especially if compared with the results for sensorineural deafness. The work of Mutton and his associates (Garvey and Mutton, 1973; Mutton and Lea, 1980) has revealed the probability of a genetic basis in some of these children. The single sex trisomies 47 XXY and 47 XYY are among the most common chromosomal abnormalities, each occurring at the rate of $^{1}/_{1000}$ male births. In a study of 121 children (including 20 girls) attending a special school for normally intelligent children with disorders of spoken language (Mutton and Lea, 1980), these forms of trisomy were detected in 3 boys, and a further 3 boys showed other anomalies.

9 The Antecedents of Disorder Communication

In human society language and communication are so closely interrelated that one might be forgiven for thinking the two are synonymous, but this is far from being the case. Individuals with normally developed linguistic skills may be singularly uncommunicative, showing little desire or perhaps ability to share ideas, thoughts and needs with those around them, and restricting their speech to the minimum which enables them to do their work, travel and buy what purchases they choose. At the other extreme there are children who though quite unable to talk, and with no "inner" verbal language at their disposal, are astonishingly effective in communicating with those around. In doing so they resort to all the various devices at their disposal, including the use of voice, facial expression, hand gesture and mime, and general bodily activity.

Case Report: **Ella**

When first seen she was 4 y 4 m old, having been referred for further assessment of her profound language disorder. Her mother had been worried about her failure to respond to sounds during the first year of life, and subsequently over her failure to talk. A number of hearing tests over the years had shown some variability but any significant degree of deafness had been excluded, and she had been admitted to a class for children with receptive language disorders. There she came under the care of a highly perceptive teacher who became convinced that she was severely deaf. She reached the conclusion that Ella was gaining her information about what was going on around her, and perhaps more bewildering, what was going to happen next, entirely visually and through her grasp of the immediate situation. She was so effective at this that her teacher wrote—"She constantly anticipates the next move. Often I cannot recall what it is that gave her the clue, but it often takes our breath away—it is as if she can mind read." She proved capable of carrying out a reliable audiogram and this revealed a loss of 100 dB at 250 Hz, 110 dB at 500 Hz, and no responses at higher frequencies to the maximum output of the audiometer. The profound level of her deafness was confirmed by electrocochleography; there was no detectable action potential at 110 dB for wide band clicks. Despite this degree of hearing loss she was an immensely communicative child. The extent of her involvement in all that was going on has already been described. At an interpersonal level she conveyed her ideas and wishes in a way which was so graphic it was almost bizarre, and it was this which no doubt mislead some of those who had seen her to conclude that she was a severely disturbed child. The truth was the reverse of this; she adopted every means at her disposal to interact with those around her. Her exaggerated facial expressions, the posturing of her body, her use of gestures of the hands and fingers, and the communicative "dances" she used were all astonishingly well-observed caricatures of the way she saw adults and children use body-language to accompany their verbal utterances.

The ability, or at least the intention and will, to communicate is far from being adjusted to a uniform level, and there are marked variations between individuals. This individual variation may be clearly apparent even within the brothers and sisters of a single nuclear family. The genetic and environmental factors which might account for this variation are poorly understood, but need constantly to be borne in mind when considering the problems of children with impaired spoken language. Given a certain level of hearing loss or mental subnormality or defective speech, each child will react in his or her unique way, depending upon the particular aggregate of constitutional, immediate family and other environmental factors which act upon him. It is possible to disentangle some of the threads. This will be attempted by considering first the role of the adult and especially the mother, and factors arising primarily within the child will subsequently be examined. The basic premise, which needs constantly to be borne in mind, is that the child is heir to the full range of communication skills which characterize the highly articulate human animal, and it is our reasonable and proper expectation that he will talk. This premise is unrelenting in its opposition to the facile attitude which dismisses the slow-talking child's problems as being due to laziness, or which too readily imputes an emotional origin and overlooks the astonishing power of the racial desire to communicate.

Parents

The characteristics of mother-child interaction have been considered at some length in Chapter 1, and again when describing the development of vocal behaviour, during the course of which the wealth of mutual interaction between parent and child was amply demonstrated. The very fact that mothers talk to their babies is thought by Snow (1977) to arise from the basis that they assume "conversation" is feasible in the first place, and is a reflection of their belief that babies are capable of reciprocal communication. She concludes "Maternal expectations about infants' abilities both arise from and are tested by the nature of the interaction mothers establish with their babies". The mother's attitude to her child, her expectations of what he is capable of doing and responding to, are in part the product of contemporary society and current practices in child-rearing. If the prevailing view is that the young child is essentially an inert recipient of food, physical care and incoming stimuli then many mothers will be subservient to such views. If it is considered that the first months of life provide a series of magical encounters with a physically helpless but astonishingly active and responsive individual, then the mother will behave in a very different way and encourage the father to do the same.

There will still, of course, be differences of attitude and behaviour, based on the personal characteristics of the parents themselves. This was seen in the study of individual differences made by Lieven (1978) who on the basis of two mother-daughter dyads found one mother to be highly responsive, and whose speech related closely to what her child was saying. The other was much less likely to extend and expand her child's speech, but instead tended to ignore or correct her child's utterances or reply with "ready-made" utterances which showed little involvement or interest in what had been said. It appears likely that the style of interaction which develops between a young child and his parents will have significant effects on the acquisition of non-linguistic communication skills from the very earliest months. The interest and attention shown by parents, their responsiveness and desire to spend time with their child, the willingness to be acted upon and take turns as recipient rather than constantly being in charge psychologically as well as physically, place demands on them which they are not necessarily able to fulfill. This may be because of their emotional states, personality characteristics and the attitudes they bring to child-rearing, or because of a wide variety of external pressures upon them. Combined together these factors affect the quality of interaction between the parents and their child, and the maturation and strength of the bonds which are formed.

The demands on the mother are considerable in terms of her time and emotional and physical energy if she is to give the requisite attention to her child. But the circumstances of the home may not permit, let alone encourage this level of commitment. There are the other members of the family to consider, and especially the constant demands for attention of the two year old sibling or the unrestrained physical activity of her four-year-old, and the meeting, collecting and taking of the older children to school quite apart from cooking, cleaning and shopping. It may be essential for her to work during part of the day in order to supplement the inadequate family income, or to work full time, especially if it is a one-parent family. Just as real as the physical limitations on her time are the emotional and other constraints which limit and distort her interaction. A mother not infrequently admits that she showed little interest in her child because she was ill, or was seriously preoccupied with the illness of an older child or some other member of the family. Depression is a well-recognized feature of the first few weeks and months after delivery, and this may be exacerbated by domestic crises over marital relationships or by financial or housing problems. The remarkably high prevalence of impoverished language in pre-school children, especially in inner-city areas, is as much a condemnation of the attitudes of society and of community provision for financially stringent young families, as it is an accurate indication of the capabilities of the mother. All these problems result in some element of deprivation of the child, in relation to the amount of time that is spent with him and in the quality of interaction or as it is frequently referred to, the amount of stimulation he receives. In his study of maternal deprivation, Rutter (1972b) considers that any developmental delay consequent upon this "is due to a *lack* of stimulation and not to the *loss* of stimulation" (his italics), as might happen when a child and his mother are separated for whatever reason, and accordingly prefers the use of the term "privation" rather than "deprivation" as being a more accurate description. The latter term is preferred for the occasions when distress is caused by separation from those with whom the child has already formed bonds of attachment. This is not necessarily only the mother, as Rutter rightly points out. Admission of a child to hospital or to a residential nursery results in

"separation from mother *and* father *and* sibs *and* the home environment. There are no studies of the short-term effects of parental absence and the influence of the father has been greatly neglected. The author's unsystematic observations of young children in families where the father spends occasional periods away from home suggest that in many families this is as likely to lead to emotional distress as is the absence of the mother." (Rutter, 1972b, p. 48, his italics)

There can be no doubt that this is true in those young children who have formed attachment bonds with their father as well as their mother, and as was seen in Chapter 1 this occurs earlier and more frequently than was once thought.

So far we have been considering the individual factors personal to the mother (and father) and arising out of the various features of their home background. These frequently pose considerable strains on the marriage and on the child's rearing, even when the child is free from any handicap or evidence of some form of developmental delay. But the problems may be overwhelming in a family who have a child whose responsivity is outside the bounds of normal, who is totally inert or who is constantly screaming and unable to settle, who appears to show no recognition of his mother, no delight in her presence or awareness of her activity, who is slow in achieving the major milestones of development, who is unable to carry on any but the most limited form of interaction with her or none at all. The professional attitude of doctors, nurses, social workers and the various groups of specialist therapists who may become involved too readily reverts to one of adverse judgement on the capabilities of the mother as a provider of care whilst remaining oblivious of the intolerable pressures placed upon her, especially when these are compounded by refusal or inability to recognize the primary nature and extent of the child's disability. It is little wonder that many such children, and this is particularly the case when the less tangible disorders of communication and spoken language are present, are said to be delayed because of some emotional disturbance in the family. That there may be clear evidence of emotional problems is undeniable but in many instances this is to make the fundamental error of mistaking effect for cause.

The Child

Interaction, as the word itself implies, is a two-way process in which the activity of the child is crucially important in determining the subsequent course of the shared involvement. Normally the child uses a wide variety of signals to express his interest, his lessening attention or boredom, his degree of anticipation, or desire to prolong the communitive episode. It may be that the child is able to experience all these emotions but quite unable to signal them, or be obliged to signal them in ways which his mother is unable to detect. As Mittler (1976) says, "whenever two organisms meet their reciprocal gestures must be mutually synchronized and balanced in a most delicate way before communication can occur". The normal child is both active in seeking the initiative in setting up an interaction, and responsive to the overtures of his mother when she does the same; and his reactions provide a source of information to the mother on how the interaction is progressing. This mutual process can be damaged or fail to start in the first case for a wide variety of reasons. The child may have a severe visual impairment and so be unable to detect his mother's signals unless her vocal behaviour and her activity in touching him, picking him up and so on are able to convey the same intentions she would normally convey through her changing facial expression and movements of her head and body. His mother may find this lack of response very disturbing because she is receiving too little feedback from his facial, hand and other movements. In the same way an autistic child abruptly disturbs the flow of his mother's communitive activity when he turns his head and eyes away. Mahoney (1975) considers that the potential non-verbal communication difficulty of autistic and mentally retarded children may not only impede language development by increasing the difficulty of the children's task in detecting the intention of the speaker, but may also interfere with the feedback system which provides the mother with the information necessary for regulating the complexity of her own language. Prior to the appearance of language itself there may well be delay in the development of the skills which are the essential antecedents of spoken language such as these interpersonal factors.

Mitchell (1976) has developed what might be called a response-tree to study more precisely the points at which interaction sequences may alternate or be disrupted. The initial overture made by one of the mother-child pair may be followed with appropriate verbal, vocal or other activity; this may be followed up by a new demand being made or the interaction may cease. Alternatively, the initial demand is not followed, in which case it may be repeated in the same form, or it may be emphasized verbally or with non-verbal cues added; this renewed demand may in its turn be followed or not followed and so on. We need to make greater use of this type of procedure in elucidating the ways in which mother-child interactions go wrong; once it is possible to identify the moments when the interaction has failed to pursue the expected course, it becomes possible to identify the reasons for the apparent failure, and put it on a quantitative basis.

Patterns of Disordered Interaction

Wing and Gould (1979) classified the patterns of social interaction in 132 severely retarded children under four headings. *Social aloofness* was the most severe impairment, some of the children showing no interest in others at any time, whilst others might make approaches for things they wanted, and some might enjoy the physical contact of cuddling or chasing but with no interest in the social aspects of the contact. *Passive interaction* described the behaviour of children who did not show any spontaneous efforts at social contact but who were amenable to the approaches of others. *Active, but odd interaction* included children who did make spontaneous approaches, mostly to adults but also to other children, but in whom there was no feeling for the needs and ideas of others, and who continued to pursue their own activities even in the face of active discouragement. *Appropriate interaction* covered those whose social interactions were appropriate for their mental age, and who enjoyed social contact for its own sake. They would resort to eye contact, facial expression and gesture to indicate their interest, and attempt to join in conversation. The results of the study show that the most notable feature of the association between mental retardation and social impairment was the correlation between severity of retardation and the proportion of children who were socially impaired. The lower the level of intelligence, the more likely it was that the social impairment would take the form of aloofness and indifference. Their study also confirms that it is possible to find children who are severely retarded, but with social reactions appropriate to their mental age. One finds this frequently gives rise to the assertion that a particular child cannot be retarded because of the quality of his interaction and sociability; it is curiously difficult to bring oneself to realize that he is behaving, say, like a normally sociable fourteen-months-old rather than a child of 3 years.

The patterns of communicative behaviour were examined in a rather different way in the personal group of 315 children. Having established on the three-point scale previously referred to the child's levels of ability for verbal comprehension, cognitive function, and hearing, and for language production and speech, it was possible to construct a series of profiles. Twenty eight such profiles were identified, the number being reduced from 51 by coalescing the two subgroups in which the only difference was the degree of speech impairment, *i.e.* moderate and severe. Each of these 28 clinical profiles was considered to be a syndrome of language disorder (Martin, 1980). Communicative function was assessed both on the behaviour of the child and his family background, since it must inevitably be an amalgam of the two components. A child with severe impairment of attachment and interaction arising perhaps from an intrauterine rubella infection will have the severity of his impairment diminished in the cradle of a caring and stable family, whilst a child with a relatively mild problem of verbal expression may develop severe problems of interpersonal communication if his family mishandles his difficulty. There is an urgent necessity for more precise ways of formulating and assesssing such components. In the present instance such features were noted as the child's ability to relate to others, the quality of this relation, his cooperation or participation, and his desire or intent to communicate; and the parents' attitude to his disability, the quality of the environment provided by them in the less material aspects of child-rearing, the stability of the home in terms of marital relationships, separation from parents, number of home-moves and so on. These items were scored whenever information was available, and as further visits for therapy and supervision of progress provided more information. In the absence of detailed home reports on all but a few families, it is necessary to adopt some sort of system such as this so that it might be as objective and non-judgemental as possible.

The relationship between the different syndromes and communicative function assessed in this way is summarized in Table 9.1.

Table 9.1. *Syndromes of language disorder, grouped according to the impairment of function, showing the numbers of children with impaired communicative function*

Category of language disorder syndrome	Number of children	Number with impaired communicative function	Percentage
1 Whole series	315	103	33
2 Impaired verbal expression (speech and/or language; with normal hearing, non-verbal and verbal comprehension)	76	8	11
3 Impaired verbal comprehension (normal hearing and non-verbal comprehension)	31	10	32
4 Impaired hearing (normal non-verbal comprehension)	110	29	26
5 Impaired non-verbal comprehension (normal hearing)	68	39	57
6 Combined impairment of hearing and non-verbal comprehension	30	16	53

It may be seen that the various features of emotional disturbance, interaction with others, non-participation and so on, as modified by the attitudes and reactions of the child's parents, show clear differences between the major sub-groupings of language disorder. The group with impairment of language and speech production reveals the lowest number of children with associated effects on the non-verbal features of interpersonal communication. In the majority this arises out of frustration in not being able to convey to their parents the particular thoughts and observations they wish to share. Fortunately it is a characteristic of human nature that most people seek hard to understand and extract meaning from utterances directed to them, and it is probably this which determines the relatively low incidence of impairment of non-verbal communication skills. Many such children circumvent their deficits of spoken language and poor intelligibility by spontaneously developing a system of manual signs, which they can use in an astonishingly graphic way to communicate their meaning. In such children it is possible to gain an insight into their language development by questioning the parents on the number and range of signs or "hand-mimes" which the child uses, and the number he can put together in his "utterances". Once a child can begin to communicate effectively, either in this way or as his speech becomes intelligible to others, and he can begin to talk at the appropriate rate and level of complexity which will convey his thoughts, his frustration diminishes rapidly. It is astonishing to find a considerable body of opinion which asserts that children who behave in this intelligent and effective way are lazy, and resort to signing because it is easier for them than talking. The corollary of this line of thought is that the child must be stopped signing otherwise he will never talk. Nothing could be further from the truth.

Case Report: **Vivian**

She was seen first at age 9 y 3 m because of a possible underlying language disorder, since she was making very poor progress in learning to talk. Her mother had suspected deafness from the time she was 6 m old as there was no vocalization in comparison with her twin sister. She had been born at 36 weeks, birth weight was 1820 g (4 lbs), she had to be intubated and tube fed. She did not suck for six months and was a very slow feeder, but there were no feeding problems after 1 y and she was walking unaided by 14 m. A number of hearing tests were carried out from 8 m; a hearing aid was provided at 5 y and she was admitted to a unit for partial hearing children. She was not saying any words. When seen she had achieved a total vocabulary of 30 words and was trying to join words in the simpler forms of two-word utterance such as "boy ... ball". She would amplify meaning by additional gesture and she spontaneously used a great deal of mimicry and gesture. She was a friendly child, anxious—indeed desperate—to communicate and would sometimes burst into tears when her family failed to understand her. Even with her aids on it was necessary to shout to gain her attention, and when talking to her face to face she was only able to recognize one word at a time. She was greatly helped by the smallest amount of gesture, and was unable to carry out a simple request without its help. Her auditory threshold was a uniform 80 dB across the frequency range in the better ear, which with her body-worn aid set at her optimum setting was improved to 50 dB. At this time she changed her school to a unit where the teaching staff employed the British deaf sign system and finger spelling to complement the spoken word. When seen six months later there had been a great increase in her vocabulary and she was able to understand more complex requests when these were spoken to her. Instead of a vocabulary limited to some nouns, people's names and one or two verbs, she understood and used adjectives and prepositions also. She was more relaxed in herself and more assured, was always willing to try and talk to convey her news and was using three-word utterances spontaneously, though the syntax was often wrong. There had also been a marked improvement in her written language. Her performance IQ on the Wechsler scale was 107 and her verbal comprehension, when assessed formally on the Reynell Developmental Language Scale was at the 3 y 6 m level, showing a gain of nearly two years in the six months since her first visit.

Children resort to hand, face and any other signalling procedures they can devise to convey their meaning, and in doing so reveal the intensity of their desire to communicate. The ideas and observations in their heads must be transmitted somehow, and if the functioning of their speech apparatus proves to be inadequate to their purpose they develop another channel of communication. Once they have effective control of spoken language they always discard the manual channel, and in doing so assert the fundamental truth that we are born to speak.

Mutism of Emotional Origin

In some children the desire to communicate is overshadowed by certain characteristics of personality and they become silent, refusing to talk in the presence of strangers. The condition is sometimes labelled "elective mutism" and in a certain sense the term is accurate but it fails to convey the nature of the child's problem. In the majority of children seen personally, it is possible to demonstrate some deficit of speech or expressive language which renders the child difficult to understand to all except his familiars. Such children, because of a heightened sense of self-awareness, know only too well that they sound strange to strangers and will encounter difficulties in talking with them, so they adopt an appropriate way out of their difficulties. The stratagem is a manifestation of impaired production of spoken language in a particular personality, and as the child's speech improves so he begins more readily to talk to his teacher at school and to the various other adults with whom he comes in contact. There are of course children in whom contact with non-familiar adults is too daunting to permit them to talk readily who have no difficulties with spoken language, but the possibility of defective speech needs always to be borne in mind until it can confidently be excluded.

There are a very small number of children in whom one has to consider that there is a true primary disorder of emotional behaviour which affects their interpersonal relations and is associated with a severe language disorder.

Case Report: **Jennifer**

She was developing normally in every respect until the age of 3 y when various members of the family contracted an influenza-like illness and she became severely ill, developing some form of encephalitis. She was very withdrawn and unresponsive so that she appeared to be deaf, her understanding for speech deteriorated and she completely lost her own speech; she was in addition extremely uncooperative at home, and difficult to handle. When seen first at the age of 5 y 10 m she showed no verbal comprehension or speech; vocalization was limited to an occasional humming sound and one or two other sounds which had a word-like quality. Hearing was normal, and this was confirmed by electrocochleography; there were no specific neurological signs. Her visuo-motor, performance skills were normal and she could draw and model in an expressive and well-developed manner. The most notable feature was her very limited interaction with others. She was extremely uncomfortable with any more than one or two people at a time, and rapidly became upset as the numbers of people—children or adults—increased around her; and she was unable to meet a person's gaze or to tolerate direct relationships with all but a very limited number of people. With these few there was a small amount of physical interaction by simple pulling and pushing, and a suggestion of affection. Beause of her normal visual skills it was felt that introduction of the Paget Gorman sign system, used by all the teaching, therapy and nursery-care staff in the Unit, would encourage communication but it had no effect for several years. Regular psychotherapy at this time failed to produce any alteration in her behaviour. By the time she was 8 y she was becoming more mature and relaxed with some understanding of sharing but there was no development of verbal understanding or expression either by speech or manually though she occasionally used her voice. At 9½ y her mother described her as being more of a companion; she was easier to communicate with and liked people around but signing was limited to labelling a few objects and there were no spoken words. She did respond with pleasure to the notice her parents took of her, but never made any spontaneous efforts to elicit this. Her mother felt it was as if she did not want or need to communicate. At school, where there was a particularly sensitive environment to her problems, her head teacher commented that she was by now much more aware of the adults who were most important to her. She had begun to tolerate games with children she knew, but strangers and other children were ignored. By her eleventh birthday she was more outgoing, was beginning to make positive attempts to develop friendships with children around her, was showing some understanding of social situations and wanting to participate in groups.

In her, it was as if the fundamental basis of interpersonal behaviour and communication, the communitive instinct itself, had been almost completely destroyed by her illness and was only beginning to recover many years later, shown by her increasing desire and ability to communicate and her very gradually widening social awareness.

Hearing Loss

It is perhaps surprising, and certainly distressing, to find that at least one quarter of the deaf children were showing evidence of impaired non-verbal communicative function. It will be recalled that moderate impairment of hearing covered the range from 40 dB to 75 dB, and yet in the 54 out of 110 children in this sub-group there was the same percentage of children (26%) with impaired communicative function as for the 56 with severe deafness. This proportion falls to that for the children with problems of expressive language disorder (category 2 in Table 9.1) if one only considers the deaf children, both moderate and severe, in whom verbal comprehension is good. The communicative problems of these children clearly does not correlate with the degree of hearing loss. The limited evidence available from this series suggests that the child's ability to understand what is said to him and to acquire language which he can use to supplement internal thought, might prove to be the significant factor in reducing his difficulties of interpersonal behaviour. Whether or not there is any truth in such a generalization, it is clear that the child with expressive difficulties is less disturbed in his relations with others than the child with impaired comprehension. In the absence of such evidence it might have been argued that children with expressive problems would experience greater frustration and emotional upset.

That such problems should arise is hardly to be wondered at, and they begin long before verbal language begins to appear in the course of normal development. Hearing is a highly sensitive instrument for monitoring the verbal behaviour of the child's mother, even if the sounds convey no linguistic message for him. The varying contours of intonation, which as we have seen, are perceived very early on, the variations of loudness, the rhythms of speech conveyed by the stress, the pulsed syllabic structure, and the modulation of rate and temporal patterning, are vital precursors of speech. As control of these is achieved the child is able to imitate other, more specifically pre-linguistic features such as patterned groups of consonant- and vowel-like sounds which become perceptually salient to him in the months leading up to the first appearance of words. This is all achieved by a highly sophisticated and long-continued use of sound games played between mother and child in which the basic rules of conversation, the turn-taking and turn-relinquishing devices, are elaborated. The deaf child is denied all of this, and in no way can it be overcome by the device of fitting him with a hearing aid. This is to overlook all the antecedents of speech, language and verbal communication skills. It can be seen that the deaf child's problems are not restricted to language acquisition as such, crucially important though it is, and his problems in communication are a reflection of this.

Mental Handicap

It might be reasoned that the prevalence of disordered communication would be lower in the mentally subnormal child, in comparison with children showing impaired comprehension or expression of language or in the deaf, since their overall awareness would be reduced in proportion to their cognitive and language deficits. That this is not the case is shown in Table 9.1 with more than half this group of children having impaired communicative function, over and above that appropriate to their mental age. This supports the findings of Wing and Gould (1979) referred to above. The problem is not a straightforward one since there is a sharp contrast between the communicative behaviour of a retarded child who is labelled autistic and another child with the same degree of retardation who say, exhibits Down's syndrome. It is customary to separate social and cognitive functions and this division was adopted in earlier chapters. Such a division is convenient for purposes of discussion but ultimately is misleading. The innate communitive instinct of the young child to be with his mother (and to continue in a necessarily different form the intimate attachment which existed for the first nine months of life from conception), must be mediated and modified through the sensory information which he receives through his eyes, ears, nose, mouth, hands and other parts of the body. All this data has to be organized into a coherent and meaningful representation of the world around and especially of his mother. The discovery of his mother as a person does not depend on some mystical coupling; the metaphysical umbilical cord which unites them after birth has its own developmental history, and this history is that of the growth of attachment considered in Chapter 1. Cognitive processes are essential. If the child is unable to perceive his mother as a person, or himself as a (personal) object among other objects, human and inanimate, then inevitably his ability and his motivation to communicate will be impaired.

The Nature of Language Production

In an earlier chapter it was noted (p. 119) that some writers, notably Chomsky as supported by McNeill and others, considered the task of language acquisition by the child to be so daunting and mysterious that the necessity for an innate Language Acquisition Device was inescapable. The alternative view, based on an understanding of the cognitive bases of language, does however receive considerable support, typified by Bruner (1967, 1974) and Sinclair-de Zwart (1971, 1973) amongst many who favour the viewpoint expressed by Piaget, that language is explicable in terms of cognitive development. The various arguments for and against either position are summarized in Moerk (1977). One's own conception of language development in the child, arrived at by a very different process and based on clinical experience of the numerous patterns of disturbed language acquisition, has clearly been in favour of the cognitive approach. Nevertheless, at the outset of writing, one retained a furtive suspicion that, though the Chomskian view was untenable in any nontrivial sense, there would come a point when it would be necessary to postulate an innate language acquisition device to explain what would otherwise prove to be inexplicable features of disordered verbal comprehension. The time has come when the question of the possibility of its existence must be asked formally. And the formal answer must be that there is no evidence, either from consideration of the course of normal development or from consideration of the pathology of spoken language in the child, to support the concept of a language acquisition device. Given the normal processes of child-rearing, with all the ordinary opportunities of personal interaction, and combined with the sensory and cognitive equipment of the normal child, the acquisition of language is a natural consequence. The corollary of this conclusion is that the more closely one looks at children with disordered comprehension of language the more likely one is to find evidence of a cognitive deficit. There is inevitably an element of doubt in some children about the nature, extent and significance of such a cognitive deficit, which it must be noted is postulated to be the cause and not the effect of the linguistic deficit.

Let us suppose, for argument's sake, that various types of cognitive structure can be arranged along a scale, with the language acquisition device at the extreme right hand end. In children with disorders of verbal comprehension it is maintained that there is no point along the scale where one could say with any measure of confidence—further to the right of this point we shall find no evidence of cognitive deficit, therefore the language acquisition device exists in its own right as a neurolinguistic reality, and it can be damaged solely and specifically.

If we look at the production of spoken language, the position is very different. We can use the same argument and postulate a scale of disorder with a specific language production device at the extreme right hand end, and say the distance along the scale between the last recognizable cause or antecedent of disordered spoken language and the language production device is so great we must logically entertain the necessity of its existence. In order to appreciate the point, it is necessary to accept that "language" is a system, an entity, a specific human activity or behaviour which exists in its own right, dependent upon but distinct from cognitive and communicative activity, and having its own special systems components and rules. If the possibility of a language production "device" (or preferably "system") is accepted, certain difficulties arise, not the least being the essential asymetry it introduces between comprehension and the production of language. But this is no real obstacle, and much that is otherwise inexplicable begins to make sense. For example, there are surprisingly large numbers of children in whom language production is specifically and unaccountably delayed, in whom verbal comprehension is age appropriate, and in whom there is no evidence of disturbed neuromotor function in the control of the speech apparatus. Because of the cohesive bond between language and speech, many speech disorders will themselves be identifiable as disorders of the language production system. The temporal relationships between the development of the understanding and the production of speech become meaningful rather than having to be taken for granted, and are perhaps a manifestation of the way in which language appeared.

It is likely that in the course of pre-human evolution one of the features which established a particular tool-using species as mankind was a stepwise jump in the ability to communicate. The intense desire, part cognitive, part emotional, to make sense of the world is a racial characteristic the origins of which are demonstrable from earliest infancy. There is a similar intensity of desire to communicate our understanding of the objective world and the world of interpersonal relations. This also is demonstrable from earliest infancy. It is submitted that at some period in time there was a catalytic fusion between the two, the full consequences of which have yet to be discovered. Out of this fusion arose the ability to construct patterned and rule-ordered sounds which signify the internalized images or representations of our environment and our reactions to it. Spoken language permits these to become externalized once again. So it is that they can be shared with other members of the community, both in the immediate present, and in continuity from generation to generation, through the initial agency of mother and child. We might account for the origins of our species by saying with Saint John (Chapter 1, Verse 1) in a somewhat different context—

"In the beginning was the Word".

References

Ambrose, J. A. (1961): The Development of the Smiling Response in Infancy. In: Determinants of Infant Behaviour (Foss, B. M., ed.). New York: Wiley.

Bartak, L., Rutter, M., Cox, A. (1975): A comparative study of infantile autism and specific developmental receptive language disorder: I. The children. Brit. J. Psychiat. *126*, 127–145.

Bayley, N. (1935): The development of motor skills in the first three years. Monogr. Soc. Res. Ch. Develop. *1*.

Beagley, H. A. (1980): Electrophysiological tests of hearing. In: Audiology and Audiological Medicine (Beagley, H. A., ed.). Oxford: University Press.

Bennet, M. J. (1979): Trials with the auditory response cradle. 1. Neonatal responses to auditory stimuli. Brit. J. Audiol. *13*, 125–134.

Berlyne, D. E. (1954): Comments on relations between Piaget's theory and S–R theory. Soc. Res. Child Develop. Monogr. *27*, 127–131.

Birns, B., Blank, M., Bridger, W. H., Escalona, S. (1965): Behavioural inhibition in neonates produced by auditory stimuli. Child Develop. *36*, 639–645.

Bloom, L. (1970): Language Development: Form and Function in Emerging Grammars. Cambridge, Mass.: M. I. T. Press.

Bloom, L. (1971): Why not pivot grammar? J. Sp. Hear. Dis. *36*, 40–45.

Bower, T. G. R. (1977): A Primer of Infant Development. San Francisco: W. H. Freeman.

Bowlby, J. (1958): The nature of the child's tie to his mother. Int. J. Psychoanal. *39*, 350–373.

Braine, M. D. S. (1963): The ontogeny of English phrase structure: the first phrase. Lang. *39*, 1–13.

Broadbent, D. E. (1958): Perception and Communication. London: Pergamon.

Bronson, G. (1974): The postnatal growth of visual capacity. Child Develop. *45*, 873–890.

Brown, R. (1973): A First Language. The Early Stages. Cambridge, Mass.: Harvard University Press.

Bruner, J. S. (1957): Going Beyond the Information Given. In: Contemporary Approaches to Cognition (Bruner, J. S., *et al.*, eds.). Cambridge, Mass.: Harvard University Press.

Bruner, J. S. (1967): The Ontogenesis of Symbols. In: To Honour Roman Jakobson. Essays on the occasion of his Seventieth Birthday. The Hague: Mouton.

Bruner, J. S. (1973): Beyond the Information Given. London: Allen and Unwin.

Bruner, J. S. (1974): Nature and Uses of Immaturity. In: The Growth of Competence (Connolly, K., Bruner, J. S., eds.). London: Academic Press.

Bruner, J. S. (1975): The Ontogenesis of speech acts. J. Child Lang. *2*, 1–19.

C. E. C. (Commission of the European Community) (1979): Childhood Deafness in the European Community. EUR 6413. Luxembourg: C. E. C.

Chomsky, N. (1965): Aspects of the Theory of Syntax. Cambridge, Mass.: M. I. T. Press.

Clark, E. V. (1974): Some Aspects of the Conceptual Basis for First Language Acquisition. In: Language Perspectives — Acquisition, Retardation and Intervention (Schiefelbusch, R. L., Lloyd, L. L., eds.). London: Macmillan.
Clifton, R. K., Graham, F. K., Hatton, H. M. (1968): Newborn heart rate response and response habituation as a function of stimulus duration. J. Exp. Child Psychol. *6*, 265—278.
Condon, W. S. (1975): Speech Makes Babies Move. In: Child Alive (Lewin, R., ed.). London: Temple Smith.
Condon, W. S., Sander, L. W. (1974): Neonate movement is synchronized with adult speech: interactional participation and language acquisition. Science *183*, 99.
Conrad, R. (1964): Acoustic confusions in immediate memory. Brit. J. Psychol. *55*, 75—84.
Conrad, R. (1972): Short term memory in the deaf: a test for speech coding. Brit. J. Psychol. *63*, 173—180.
Conrad, R. (1979): The Deaf School Child; Language and Cognitive Function. London: Harper and Row.
Cooper, J., Moodley, M., Reynell, J. (1978): Helping Language Development. London: Arnold.
Crystal, D. (1973): Non-segmental phonology in language acquisition: a review of the issues. Lingua *32*, 1—45.
Crystal, D. (1975): The English Tone of Voice. London: Arnold.
Crystal, D., Fletcher, P., Gorman, M. (1978): The Grammatical Analysis of Language Disability. London: Arnold.
Dale, P. S. (1976): Language Development. Hinsdale, Ill.: Dryden Press.
Dearborn, G. V. N. (1910): Moto-Sensory Development: Observations of the First Three Years of a Child. Baltimore: Warwick and York. (Quoted in Eisenberg, R. B., 1976.)
Desmond, M. M., Rudolph, A. J., Phitaksphraiwan, P. (1966): The transitional care nursery: a mechanism of a preventive medicine. Paed. Clin. North Amer. *13*, 651—668.
de Villiers, J. G., de Villiers, P. A. (1974): Competence and performance in child language: are children really competent to judge? J. Child Lang. *1*, 11—22.
Dore, J. (1975): Holophrases, speech acts and language universals. J. Child Lang. *2*, 21—40.
Drillien, C. M. (1977): Developmental Assessment and Development Screening. In: Neurodevelopmental Problems in Early Childhood (Drillien, C. M., Drummond, M. B., eds.). Oxford: Blackwell.
Edwards, M. L. (1974): Perception and production in child phonology: the testing of four hypotheses. J. Child Lang. *2*, 205—219.
Eimas, P. D. (1974): Linguistic Processing of Speech by Young Infants. In: Language Perspectives — Acquisition, Retardation and Intervention (Schiefelbusch, R. L., Lloyd, L. L., eds.). London: Macmillan.
Eimas, P. D., Siqueland, E. R., Jusczyk, P., Vigorito, J. (1971): Speech perception in infants. Science *171*, 303—306.
Eisenberg, R. B. (1965): Auditory behaviour in the human neonate. I. Methodologic problems and the logical design of research procedures. J. Aud. Res. *5*, 159—177.
Eisenberg, R. B. (1976): Auditory Competence in Early Life. The Roots of Communicative Behaviour. Baltimore: University Park Press.
Eisenson, J., Auer, T., Irwin, J. (1963): The Psychology of Communication. New York.
Elliott, J., Connolly, K. (1974): Hierarchical Structure in Skill Development. In: The Growth of Competence (Connolly, K., Bruner, J., eds.). London: Academic Press.
Fantz, R. L. (1961): The origin of form perception. Scient. Amer. *204*, 66—72.
Fantz, R. L. (1965): Visual perception from birth as shown by pattern selectivity. Ann. N. Y. Acad. Sci. *118*, 793—814.
Foley, J. (1977): Cerebral Palsy — Physical Aspects. In: Neurodevelopmental Problems in Early Childhood (Drillien, C. M., Drummond, M. B., eds.). Oxford: Blackwell.
Fourcin, A. J. (1978): Acoustic Patterns and Speech Acquisition. In: The Development of Communication (Waterson, N., Snow, C., eds.). Chichester: Wiley.
Fourcin, A. J. (1979): Personal communication.
Fraser, G. R. (1976): The Causes of Profound Deafness in Childhood. Baltimore: Johns Hopkins University Press.
Fry, D. B. (1958): Experiments in the perception of stress. Lang. and Sp. *1*, 126—152.
Garvey, M., Mutton, D. E. (1973): Sex chromosome aberrations and speech development. Arch. Dis. Child. *48*, 937—941.

Gibson, W. P. R. (1978): Essentials of Clinical Electric Response Audiometry. Edinburgh: Churchill Livingstone.

Goren, C., Sarty, M., Wu, P. (1975): Visual following and pattern discrimination of face-like stimuli by newborn infants. Pediat. *56*, 544—549.

Gratch, G. (1976): On levels of awareness of objects in infants and students thereof. Merrill-Palmer Quart. *22*, 157—176. Reprinted in: Early Cognitive Development (Oares, J., ed.) (1979): London: Groom Helm and Open University Press.

Gratch, G., Landers, W. F. (1971): Stage IV of Piaget's theory of infants' object concepts: a longitudinal study. Child Develop. *42*, 359—372.

Greenfield, P. M. (1978): Informativeness, Presupposition and Semantic Choice in Single-Word Utterances. In: The Development of Communication (Waterson, N., Snow, C., eds.). Chichester: Wiley.

Greenfield, P. M., Smith, J. H. (1976): The Structure of Communication in Early Language Development. New York: Academic Press.

Griffiths, P. (1972): Developmental Aphasia: an Introduction. London: Invalid Children's Aid Association.

Grollenberg, L. H. (1959): Shorter Atlas of the Bible. Edinburgh: Nelson.

Haaf, R. A., Bell, R. Q. (1967): A facial dimension in visual discrimination by human infants. Child Develop. *38*, 893—899.

Haith, M. M. (1976): Visual Competence in Early Infancy. In: Handbook of Sensory Physiology, Vol. 8 (Held, R., Leibowitz, H., Teuber, H. L., eds.). Berlin-Heidelberg-New York: Springer.

Haith, M. M., Campos, J. J. (1977): Human infancy. Ann. Rev. Psychol. *28*, 251—293.

Haller, M. W. (1932): The reactions of infants to changes in the intensity and pitch of pure tone. J. Genet. Psychol. *40*, 162—180.

Hamburger, V. (1977): The developmental history of the motor neurone. Neurosci. Res. Progr. Bull. *15*, April Supplement.

Hobsbaum, A., Mittler, P. (1971): Sentence Comprehension Test. University of Manchester: Hester Adrian Research Centre.

Howe, C. J. (1976): The meanings of two-word utterances in the speech of young children. J. Child Lang. *3*, 29—47.

Ingram, T. T. S. (1972): The Classification of Speech and Language Disorders in Young Children. In: The Child with Delayed Speech (Rutter, M., Martin, J. A. M., eds.). (Spastics International Medical Publications.) London: Heinemann.

Jakobson, R., Fant, C. G. M., Halle, M. (1952): Preliminaries to Speech Analysis: The Distinctive Features and Their Correlates. Cambridge, Mass.: M. I. T. Press.

Jakobson, R., Halle, M. (1968): Phonology in Relation to Phonetics. In: Manual of Phonetics (Malmberg, B., ed.). Amsterdam: North-Holland.

Johns, D. F., LaPointe, L. L. (1976): Neurogenic Disorders of Output Processing: Apraxia of Speech. In: Studies in Neurolinguistics, Vol. 1 (Whitaker, H., Whitaker, H. A., eds.). New York: Academic Press.

Kearsley, R. B. (1973): The newborn's response to auditory stimulation: a demonstration of orienting and defensive behaviour. Child Develop. *44*, 582—590.

Keen, R. E. (1964): Effects of auditory stimuli on sucking behaviour in the human neonate. J. Exper. Child Psychol. *1*, 348—354.

Klaus, M. H., Kennell, J. H. (1976): Maternal-Infant Bonding. Saint Louis: Mosby.

Lackner, J. R. (1968): A developmental study of language behaviour in retarded children. Neuropsychologia *6*, 301—320.

Lenard, H. G., van Bernuth, H., Hutt, S. J. (1969): Acoustic evoked responses in newborn infants: the influence of pitch and complexity of the stimulus. Electroencephal. Clin. Neurophysiol. *27*, 121 to 127.

Leopold, W. F. (1947): Speech Development of a Bilingual Child, Vol. 2: Sound Learning in the First Two Years. Evanston, Ill.: North-Western University Press.

Leventhall, A., Lipsitt, L. P. (1964): Adaptation, pitch discrimination and sound localization in the neonate. Child Develop. *35*, 759—767.

Lieven, E. V. M. (1978): Conversations Between Mothers and Young Children: Individual Differences and Their Possible Implication for the Study of Language Learning. In: The Development of Communication (Waterson, N., Snow, C., eds.). Chichester: Wiley.

Lorenz, K. Z. (1952): King Solomon's Ring. London: Methuen.
Lorenz, K. Z. (1969): Innate Bases of Learning. In: On the Biology of Learning (Pribram, K. H., ed.). New York: Harcourt, Brace and World.
Lynip, A. W. (1951): The use of magnetic devices in the collection and analysis of the preverbal utterances of an infant. Genet. Psychol. Monogr. *44*, 221–262.
McKay, E. (1977): Mental Retardation. In: Neurodevelopmental Problems in Early Childhood (Drillien, C. M., Drummond, M. B., eds.). Oxford: Blackwell.
MacKeith, R. C., Rutter, M. (1972): A Note on the Prevalence of Speech and Language Disorders. In: The Child with Delayed Speech (Rutter, M., Martin, J. A. M., eds.). (Spastics International Medical Publications.) London: Heinemann.
McKenzie, B., Day, R. H. (1971): Orientation discrimination in infants: a comparison of visual fixation and operant training. J. Exp. Psychol. *11*, 366–375.
McNeill, D. (1970): The Acquisition of Language: the Study of Developmental Psycholinguistics. New York: Harper and Row.
Mahoney, G. J. (1975): Ethological approach to delayed language acquisition. Amer. J. Ment. Def. *80*, 139–148.
Martin, J. A. M. (1963): Congenital laryngeal stridor. J. Laryngol. Otol. *77*, 290–298.
Martin, J. A. M. (1980): Syndrome Delineation in Communication Disorders. In: Language and Language Disorders in Childhood (Hersor, L. A., Berger, M., Nicol, A. R., eds.). Oxford: Pergamon.
Martin, J. A. M., Martin, D. E. (1973): Auditory perception. Brit. Med. J. *2*, 459–461.
Menyuk, P. (1971): The Acquisition and Development of Language. Englewood Cliffs, N. J.: Prentice-Hall.
Miller, G. A., Nicely, P. E. (1955): An analysis of perceptual confusions among some consonants. J. Acoust. Soc. Amer. *27*, 338–352.
Mitchell, D. (1976): Parent-Child Interaction in the Mentally Handicapped. In: Language and Communication in the Mentally Handicapped (Berry, P., ed.). London: Arnold.
Mittler, P. (1972): Language Development and Mental Handicaps. In: The Child with Delayed Speech (Rutter, M., Martin, J. A. M., eds.). (Spastics International Medical Publications.) London: Heinemann.
Mittler, P. (1976): In: Language and Communication in the Mentally Handicapped (Berry, P., ed.). London: Arnold.
Moerk, E. L. (1977): Pragmatic and Semantic Apects of Early Language Development. Baltimore: University Park Press.
Moffitt, A. R. (1971): Consonant cue perception by twenty- to twenty four-week-old infants. Child Develop. *42*, 717–732.
Morley, M. E. (1972): The Development and Disorders of Speech in Childhood, 3rd ed. Edinburgh: Churchill Livingstone.
Morse, P. A. (1972): The discrimination of speech and non-speech stimuli in early infancy. J. Exper. Child Psychol. *14*, 477–492.
Muller, E., Hollien, H., Murry, T. (1974): Perceptual responses to infant crying: identification of cry types. J. Child Lang. *1*, 89–95.
Murry, T., Amundson, P., Hollien, H. (1977): Acoustical characteristics of infant cries: fundamental frequency. J. Child Lang. *4*, 321–328.
Mutton, D. E., Lea, J. (1980): Chromosome studies of children with specific speech and language delay. Develop. Med. Child. Neurol. *22*, 588–594.
O'Connor, N., Hermelin, B. (1963): Speech and Thought in Severe Subnormality. Oxford: Pergamon Press.
Piaget, J. (1954): The Construction of Reality in the Child. (Translated by M. Cook.) London: Routledge and Kegan Paul.
Piaget, J. (1962): Play, Dreams and Imitation in Childhood. (Translated by C. Gattegno and F. M. Hodgson.) London: Routledge and Kegan Paul.
Quirk, R., Greenbaum, S., Leech, G., Swartvik, J. (1972): A Grammar of Contemporary English. London: Longman.
Rees, N. S. (1971): Bases of decision in language training. J. Sp. Hear. Dis. *36*, 283–304.
Rees, N. S. (1973): Auditory processing factors in language disorders: the view from Procrustes bed. J. Sp. Hear. Dis. *38*, 304–315.

Reynell, J. (1969): Test Manual; Reynell Developmental Language Scales. Slough: National Foundation for Educational Research.

Ricks, D. (1972): The Beginning of Vocal Communication in Infants and Autistic Children. University of London: Unpublished doctoral thesis.

Ricks, D. (1975): Vocal Communication in Pre-Verbal Normal and Autistic Children. In: Language, Cognitive Deficits and Retardation (O'Connor, N., ed.). London: Butterworths.

Ringler, N. (1978): A Longitudinal Study of Mother's Language. In: The Development of Communication (Waterson, N., Snow, C., eds.). Chichester: Wiley.

Rodgon, M. M. (1976): Single-Word Usage, Cognitive Development, and the Beginnings of Combinatorial Speech. A Study of Ten English-Speaking Children. Cambridge: University Press.

Rutter, M. (1972 a): Psychiatric Causes of language Retardation. In: The Child with Delayed Speech (Rutter, M., Martin, J. A. M., eds.). (Spastics International Medical Publications.) London: Heinemann.

Rutter, M. (1972 b): Maternal Deprivation Reassessed. Harmondsworth: Penguin Books.

Sachs, J., Truswell, L. (1978): Comprehension of two-word instructions by children in the one-word stage. J. Child Lang. *5,* 17–24.

Schaffer, H. R. (1971): The Growth of Sociability. Harmondsworth: Penguin Books.

Schaffer, H. R., Emerson, P. E. (1964): The development of social attachments in infancy. Monogr. Soc. Res. Child Develop. *29,* No. 3.

Schlesinger, I. M. (1971): Production of Utterances and Language Acquisition. In: The Ontogenesis of Grammar (Slobin, D. I., ed.). New York: Academic Press.

Sheridan, M. S. (1968): Playthings in the development of language. Health Trends. *1,* 7.

Sheridan, M. S. (1975): Children's Developmental Progress. Slough: National Foundation for Educational Research.

Sheridan, M. S. (1977): Spontaneous Play in Early Childhood. Slough: National Foundation for Educational Research.

Simmons, F. B., Russ, F. N. (1974): Automated newborn hearing screening, the Crib-o-gram. Arch. Otolaryngol. *100,* 1–7.

Sinclair, H. (1971): Sensorimotor Action Patterns as a Condition for the Acquisition of Syntax. In: Language Acquisition: Models and Methods (Huxley, R., Ingram, E., eds.). London: Academic Press.

Sinclair-de Zwart, H. (1973): Language Acquisition and Cognitive Development. In: Cognitive Development and the Acquisition of Language (Moore, T. E., ed.). New York: Academic Press.

Slater, A. M., Findlay, J. M. (1972): The measurement of fixation position in the newborn baby. J. Exper. Child Psychol. *20,* 248–273.

Slobin, D. I. (1970): Universals of grammatical development. In: Advances in Psycholinguistics (Flores d'Arcais, G. B., Levelt, W. J. M., eds.). Amsterdam: North-Holland.

Smith, M. E. (1926): An investigation of the development of the sentence and the extent of vocabulary in young children. University of Iowa Studies in Child Welfare. *3,* No. 5. (Quoted in Dale, P. S., 1976.)

Snow, C. E. (1977): The development of conversation between mothers and babies. J. Child Lang. *4,* 1 to 22.

Sroufe, L. A., Waters, E. (1976): The ontogenesis of smiling and laughter: a perspective on the organization of development in infancy. Psychol. Rev. *83,* 173–189.

Stern, C., Stern, W. (1907): Die Kindersprache: Eine psychologische und sprachtheoretische Untersuchung. Leipzig: Barth. (Quoted in Rodgon, M. M., 1976.)

Stern, D. (1974): Mother and Infant at Play: The Dyadic Interaction Involving Facial, Vocal and Gaze Behaviours. In: The Effect of the Infant on Its Caregiver (Lewis, M., Rosenblum, L., eds.). New York: Wiley.

Stern, D. (1977): The First Relationship: Infant and Mother. London: Fontana/Open Books.

Tallal, P., Piercy, M. (1973): Defects of non-verbal auditory perception in children with developmental dysphasia. Natur. *241,* 468–499.

Tallal, P., Piercy, M. (1974): Developmental aphasia; rate of auditory processing and selective impairment of consonant perception. Neuropsychol. *12,* 83–93.

Tallal, P., Piercy, M. (1975): Developmental aphasia; the perception of brief vowels and extended stop consonants. Neuropsychol. *13,* 69–74.

Tallal, P., Piercy, M. (1978): Defects of Auditory Perception in Children with Developmental Dysphasia. In: Developmental Dysphasia (Wyke, M. A., ed.). London: Academic Press.

Tinbergen, N. (1951): The Study of Instinct. Oxford: University Press.

Touwen, B. (1976): Neurological Development in Infancy. (Spastics International Medical Publications.) London: Heinemann.

Turkewitz, G., Birch, H. G., Cooper, K. K. (1972): Patterns of response to different auditory stimuli in the human newborn. Develop. Med. Child Neurol. *14*, 487–491.

Tyson, A. (ed.) (1967): Selected Letters of Beethoven. (Translated by Emily Anderson.) London: Macmillan.

Wasz-Hockert, O., Lind, J., Vuorenkoski, V., Partanen, T. J., Valanne, E. (1968): The Infant Cry: a Spectrographic and Auditory Analysis. (Spastics International Medical Publications.) London: Heinemann.

Wasz-Hockert, O., Partanen, T. J., Vuorenkoski, V., Valanne, E., Michelsson, K. (1964): The identification of specific meaning in infant vocalization. Experientia *20*, 154–155.

Watson, J. S. (1973): Smiling, cooing and "the game". Merrill-Palmer Quart. Behav. Develop. *18*, 323 to 339.

Webster, N. (1971): Third New International Dictionary of the English Language. Springfield, Mass.: Merriam.

Wheldall, K. (1976): Receptive Language Development in the Mentally Handicapped. In: Language and Communication in the Mentally Handicapped (Berry, P., ed.). London: Arnold.

Williams, P. L., Warwick, R. (1975): Functional Neuroanatomy of Man. Edinburgh: Churchill Livingstone.

Wing, L., Gould, J. (1979): Severe impairments of social interaction and associated abnormalities in children: epidemiology and classification. J. Aut. Develop. *9*, 11–29.

Wing, L., Gould, J., Yeates, S. R., Brierley, L. M. (1977): Symbolic play in severely mentally retarded and in autistic children. J. Child Psychol. Psychiat. *18*, 167–178.

Wolff, P. H. (1969): The Natural History of Crying and Other Vocalizations in Early Infancy. In: Determinants of Infant Behaviour, Vol. 4 (Foss, B. M., ed.). London: Methuen.

Worster-Drought, C., Allen, I. M. (1929): Congenital auditory imperception (congenital word-deafness) with report of case. J. Neurol. and Psychopathol. *9*, 193–208.

Subject Index

Disorders of Human Communication

Edited by
Godfrey E. Arnold, Jackson, Miss., USA
Fritz Winckel, Berlin (West)
Barry D. Wyke, London, Great Britain

Volume 1:

Hearing: Its Function and Dysfunction

By **Earl D. Schubert,** Ph. D., Professor of Hearing and Speech Sciences, Stanford University School of Medicine, Stanford, Calif.

1980. 86 figures. X, 184 pages.
ISBN 0-387-81579-1 (New York)
ISBN 3-211-81579-1 (Wien)

Volume 2:

Clinical Aspects of Dysphasia

By **Martin L. Albert,** M. D., Professor of Neurology, Boston University Medical School, Boston, Mass., **Harold Goodglass,** Ph. D., Professor of Neurology (Neuropsychology), Boston University Medical School, Boston, Mass., **Nancy A. Helm,** D. Sc., Assistant Professor of Neurology (Speech Pathology), Boston University Medical School, Boston, Mass., **Alan B. Rubens,** M. D., Associate Professor of Neurology, University of Minnesota Medical School, Minneapolis, Minn., **Michael P. Alexander,** M. D., Assistant Professor of Neurology, Boston University Medical School, Boston, Mass.

1981. 12 figures. XI, 194 pages.
ISBN 0-387-81617-8 (New York)
ISBN 3-211-81617-8 (Wien)

Volume 3:

Clinical Linguistics

By **David Crystal,** Professor of Linguistic Science, University of Reading, Reading, Great Britain

1981. 3 figures. XII, 228 pages.
ISBN 0-387-81622-4 (New York)
ISBN 3-211-81622-4 (Wien)

Springer-Verlag Wien New York

MIX
Papier aus verantwortungsvollen Quellen
Paper from responsible sources
FSC® C105338

If you have any concerns about our products,
you can contact us on
ProductSafety@springernature.com

In case Publisher is established outside the EU,
the EU authorized representative is:
Springer Nature Customer Service Center GmbH
Europaplatz 3, 69115 Heidelberg, Germany

Printed by Libri Plureos GmbH
in Hamburg, Germany